Atlas of Canine and Feline Urinalysis

Atlas of Canine and Feline Urinalysis

Theresa E. Rizzi
Oklahoma State University, Stillwater, OK

Amy Valenciano
IDEXX, Flower Mound, TX, USA

Mary Bowles
Oklahoma State University, Stillwater, OK, USA

Rick Cowell
IDEXX, Hillside Street, OK, USA

Ronald Tyler
Harlingen, TX, USA

Dennis B. DeNicola
Chief Veterinary Educator IDEXX Laboratories One IDEXX Drive Westbrook, ME, USA

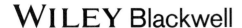

Registered Offices
John Wiley & Sons, Inc., 111 River Street, Hoboken, NJ 07030, USA

Editorial Office
111 River Street, Hoboken, NJ 07030, USA

For details of our global editorial offices, customer services, and more information about Wiley products visit us at www.wiley.com.

Wiley also publishes its books in a variety of electronic formats and by print-on-demand. Some content that appears in standard print versions of this book may not be available in other formats.

Limit of Liability/Disclaimer of Warranty
The contents of this work are intended to further general scientific research, understanding, and discussion only and are not intended and should not be relied upon as recommending or promoting scientific method, diagnosis, or treatment by physicians for any particular patient. In view of ongoing research, equipment modifications, changes in governmental regulations, and the constant flow of information relating to the use of medicines, equipment, and devices, the reader is urged to review and evaluate the information provided in the package insert or instructions for each medicine, equipment, or device for, among other things, any changes in the instructions or indication of usage and for added warnings and precautions. While the publisher and authors have used their best efforts in preparing this work, they make no representations or warranties with respect to the accuracy or completeness of the contents of this work and specifically disclaim all warranties, including without limitation any implied warranties of merchantability or fitness for a particular purpose. No warranty may be created or extended by sales representatives, written sales materials or promotional statements for this work. The fact that an organization, website, or product is referred to in this work as a citation and/or potential source of further information does not mean that the publisher and authors endorse the information or services the organization, website, or product may provide or recommendations it may make. This work is sold with the understanding that the publisher is not engaged in rendering professional services. The advice and strategies contained herein may not be suitable for your situation. You should consult with a specialist where appropriate. Further, readers should be aware that websites listed in this work may have changed or disappeared between when this work was written and when it is read. Neither the publisher nor authors shall be liable for any loss of profit or any other commercial damages, including but not limited to special, incidental, consequential, or other damages.

Library of Congress Cataloging-in-Publication Data

Names: Rizzi, Theresa E., author. | Valenciano, Amy, author. | Cowell, Rick, author. | Tyler, Ronald, author. | Bowles, Mary, 1950– author. | DeNicola, D. B., author.
Title: Atlas of canine and feline urinalysis / Dr. Theresa E. Rizzi, Dr. Amy Valenciano, Dr. Rick Cowell, Dr. Ronald Tyler, Dr. Mary Bowles, Dr. Dennis B. DeNicola.
Description: Hoboken, NJ : John Wiley & Sons Inc., 2017. | Includes index.
Identifiers: LCCN 2017006139 (print) | LCCN 2017014316 (ebook) | ISBN 9781119110354 (pbk.) | ISBN 9781119110392 (Adobe PDF) | ISBN 9781119110415 (ePub)
Subjects: LCSH: Dogs–Diseases–Diagnosis. | Cats–Diseases–Diagnosis. | Urine–Analysis. | MESH: Dog Diseases–urine | Urinalysis–veterinary | Cat Diseases–urine | Atlases
Classification: LCC SF991 .R59 2017 (ebook) | LCC SF991 (print) | NLM SF 991 | DDC 636.7089/607566–dc23
LC record available at https://lccn.loc.gov/2017014316

Cover Design: Wiley
Cover Images: Courtesy of Theresa Rizzi

Set in 10/12pt WarnockPro by Aptara Inc., New Delhi, India

Dedication

The authors would like to dedicate this Atlas to our families who supported us not only in our efforts to write the text but also in the many years spent in acquiring the knowledge to develop its content. We also dedicate this Atlas to the veterinary practitioners, technicians, diagnostic laboratory personnel, and students who strive to enhance the care of the dogs and cats that enrich people's lives.

Personal Dedications

My efforts are dedicated to Jesus Christ, Lord and Savior, and to my husband, Daniel, daughter, Avery, and son, Ty.

Amy Valenciano

To my mother who gave me my core tenants of faith, honesty and respect; my amazing wife, Reba, for her patience and support; my children – Reba, Ron, Britt, and Blake – who have made my life truly wonderful, exciting, and worthwhile; and the many exceptional colleagues who have taught, inspired and guided me – especially Roger Panciera for his mentorship and Rick Cowell for his many contributions to my development as a person and pathologist and, most of all, for his friendship through the years.

Ron Tyler

To my parents who taught me the value of honesty and instilled in me a work ethic that has served me well through the years. To my wife (Annette) and daughter (Anne) who have continually given support, meaning, and inspiration to my life. To my daughter (Rebecca) who showed me the face of true courage and taught me how to laugh and love even in the worst of times. While she lost her battle with cancer at the age of 11, her memories and life lessons will forever be remembered.

To the many outstanding veterinary clinical pathologists I have had the opportunity to learn from, especially Drs. Ronald D. Tyler, James Meinkoth, and Dennis DeNicola. To the many veterinary practitioners, residents, and students who taught me much more than I could have ever hoped to teach them and have become colleagues and friends. To IDEXX laboratories for their continued support of veterinary education.

Rick Cowell

To the many people who encouraged and assisted me during my career as a veterinary clinician and educator.

My parents who made many sacrifices to help me attain my goal of becoming a veterinarian.

My husband, John, and my children, Will and Lisa, who gave me unconditional support while experiencing many work-related interruptions in our family life.

Dr. Joe Dorner, the veterinary clinical pathologist and instructor, who first sparked my interest in clinical pathology and made me realize its importance in patient management.

Dr. Ralph Buckner, who was a wonderful mentor and role model for my development as a clinician, teacher, and human being.

The numerous contributors to the veterinary urology literature such as Drs. Carl Osborne, Jody Lulich, Stephen Dibartola, Dennis Chew, Greg Grauer, Shelly Vaden, and Joe Bartges, who helped expand my knowledge and ability to teach the subject of urology.

The students, colleagues, clients, and patients I have been privileged to know who constantly stimulated me to enhance my knowledge and skills as a clinician and a teacher.

Mary Bowles

This book is dedicated to my wife, Debbie, and son Aiden, who every day inspire me to be the person they believe I am. To my parents that instilled in me a strong work ethic and the value of integrity in all I do and to my siblings who helped me develop my sense of humor and deep sense of unconditional love. To my mentors, Drs. Rick Cowell and James Meinkoth, who gave me an opportunity many years ago and contributed to my development as a clinical pathologist; I am forever grateful. Lastly, this book is dedicated to colleagues, residents, students, and staff at Oklahoma State University who make what I do so enjoyable.

Theresa E. Rizzi

Contents

Acknowledgments   *ix*

Introduction   *1*

1   Sample Collection and Handling   *3*
Collection of Urine Samples   *3*
   Free-Catch Urine Collection   *3*
   Transurethral Catheterization   *15*
   Cystocentesis   *37*
Urine Sample Handling   *44*
   Culture   *44*

2   Initial Assessment: Physical Characteristics   *47*
Volume   *47*
Color   *47*
Clarity/Turbidity   *48*
Odor   *48*
Urine Specific Gravity   *49*

3   Urine Chemistry   *53*
Urine pH   *53*
Protein   *54*
Glucose   *60*
Ketones   *61*
Blood (Occult Blood, Heme)   *63*
Bilirubin   *64*

4   Urine Sediment   *67*
Preparation for Microscopic Examination   *67*
Casts   *67*
   Hyaline Casts   *68*
   Cellular Casts   *71*
   Granular Casts   *73*
   Waxy Casts   *78*
   Fatty Casts (Lipid Casts)   *79*
   Hemoglobin Casts   *81*

Mixed Casts   *82*
Pseudo Casts   *85*
Crystals   *86*
Crystals Associated with Urolith Formation   *86*
Crystals Not Typically Associated with Canine and Feline Urolith Formation   *120*
Drug-Induced Crystals   *130*
Cells   *131*
Transitional Epithelial Cells   *131*
Squamous Epithelial Cells   *136*
Renal Tubular (Cuboidal) Epithelial Cells   *140*
Leukocytes   *141*
Erythrocytes   *145*
Atypical (Neoplastic) Cells   *148*
Organisms   *157*
Bacteria   *157*
Fungal Hyphae   *161*
Yeast   *163*
Dioctophyma renale Ova   *165*
Capillaria plica (now *Pearsonema plica*) and *Capillaria felis cati* Ova   *166*
Microfilaria   *168*
Miscellaneous Findings and Artifacts   *169*
Pollen   *169*
Fungal Spores   *170*
Mucus   *172*
Lipid Droplets   *173*
Sperm   *174*
Air Bubbles   *176*
Starch Granules (Glove Powder)   *177*
Fiber   *178*

Reference   *181*
Index   *183*

Acknowledgments

We thank our families for their love and support. Acknowledgement and thanks are extended to the dedicated doctors, technicians, students, and staff of Oklahoma State University's Center for Veterinary Health Sciences; to John W. Bowles for photographic contributions to the many of the figures included in this Atlas; and to Wiley-Blackwell's extraordinary editors and staff.

Introduction

Urinalysis (UA) is a relatively rapid diagnostic test that provides information about the urinary system as well as other body systems, and is often performed as part of the minimum database of diagnostic tests that includes a complete blood count (CBC) and clinical biochemistry profile. Indications for performing a UA include clinical signs associated with the urinary tract, but also as part of a general health screen, in patients with systemic illness, when monitoring a response to treatment, and in screening for breed-related urinary tract disease.

There are four components to a complete UA: evaluation of the urine sample's physical characteristics, the measurement of specific gravity, assessment of chemical properties, and the microscopic examination of urine sediment. The UA, when performed in-house, should be evaluated soon after collection to eliminate artifacts that occur due to a time delay, thus emphasizing the importance of an accurate evaluation of the complete UA.

The purpose of the *Atlas of Canine and Feline Urinalysis* is to aid veterinary practitioners, veterinary technicians, veterinary students, and veterinary diagnostic laboratory personnel in the accurate collection, handling, and evaluation of canine and feline urine samples.

Atlas of Canine and Feline Urinalysis, First Edition. Theresa E. Rizzi, Amy Valenciano, Mary Bowles, Rick Cowell, Ronald Tyler, and Dennis B. DeNicola.
© 2017 John Wiley & Sons, Inc. Published 2017 by John Wiley & Sons, Inc.

1

Sample Collection and Handling

The method of urine collection and the subsequent handling of the sample can influence the interpretation of results. The following discussion is a review of urine collection and handling techniques.

Collection of Urine Samples

The three techniques for urine collection are: free-catch, catheterization, and cystocentesis. Each of these methods of collection and their associated advantages and disadvantages will be discussed. General considerations related to urine sample collection, handling, and submission, regardless of collection method, are listed in Box 1.1 (Figures 1.1–1.4).

Free-Catch Urine Collection

The free-catch method of urine collection (Box 1.2 and Figures 1.5–1.9) is often easy to perform but is dependent upon the cooperation of the patient and may be difficult to accomplish in patients with conditions producing urge incontinence. Samples are usually collected during normal voiding or by manual external compression of the urinary bladder. Normal voiding free-catch urine sampling can often be performed by the owners and does not pose a risk to the pet. The manual compression of a distended urinary bladder (Box 1.3 and Figures 1.10–1.14) may be at the convenience of the collector; however, drawbacks include

sample contamination, urinary bladder trauma, and reflux of infected urine into the ureters, kidney, and prostate. Furthermore, this technique cannot be used following a cystotomy operation and may be unpleasant in other postoperative laparotomy patients.

Collecting a midstream urine sample is preferred to minimize sample contamination; however, some contamination with cells, bacteria, and debris from the distal urethra, genital tract, and external skin and hair coat is unavoidable. Obtaining an optimal free-catch sample can be facilitated by using one container to collect the beginning of the urine stream and then changing to a second collecting container as the urine stream continues. The urine in the second container should be more representative of a true midstream sample. In some cases, a free-catch sample containing white cells, bacteria, and/or protein may be an indication to collect a subsequent patient urine sample via cystocentesis or catheterization in order to help establish the source of the abnormalities identified in the voided sample.

Sometimes a satisfactory free-catch sample cannot be obtained either during normal voiding or via manual expression, most commonly due to the pet's behavior or urge incontinence. Manual expression can be especially problematic in male cats as a result of resistance to handling and difficulty in initiating voiding due to the small diameter of the male feline urethra. Collecting urine by catheterization or cystocentesis are alternative options but not readily accomplished

Atlas of Canine and Feline Urinalysis, First Edition. Theresa E. Rizzi, Amy Valenciano, Mary Bowles, Rick Cowell, Ronald Tyler, and Dennis B. DeNicola.
© 2017 John Wiley & Sons, Inc. Published 2017 by John Wiley & Sons, Inc.

Box 1.1 **General considerations for urine sample collection, handling, and submission.**

Collection

1. Observe principles of aseptic technique as much as possible
2. Collect adequate volume (minimum of 5 mL recommended) (Figure 1.1)
3. Clean and/or sterile container provided by veterinarian preferred for collection for UA
4. Sterile container preferred for collection of sample to be cultured
5. When possible, withhold drugs and fluid administration prior to sample collection

Handling

1. Ideally UA should be performed within 60 minutes of sample collection and no longer than 6 hours following collection
2. Refrigerate and cap the sample when UA cannot be performed within 60 minutes of collection (if possible, perform the dipstick portion prior to refrigeration)
3. Refrigerated samples should be brought to room temperature prior to performing UA

Submission

1. Container submitted should identify sample as urine, be capped, and have adequate patient identification (Figure 1.2)
2. Consider using preservative tube* for storage and submission of sample for culture
3. Sample for cytologic evaluation should include one or more air-dried slides of urine sediment prepared by the blood smear or squash preparation technique along with a urine sample placed in an EDTA tube (Figure 1.3)
4. Pertinent information should be provided for samples submitted for evaluation to an outside laboratory, including patient signalment, history, and method of urine collection
5. Fasted samples submitted for evaluation frequently have increased specific gravity values, more cells and casts, and decreased pH values compared to non-fasted samples

---

UA=urinalysis
*e.g. BD Vacutainer®Culture and Sensitivity Preservative Tube. The BD 4-mL urine culture preservative tube kit includes a urine transfer straw which can be used to facilitate aspiration of urine into the tube (Figure 1.4). Use of the transfer straw is optional. Although the manufacturer recommends adding a minimum of 3 mL of patient urine for an optimum preservative to urine ratio, obtaining that amount for urine from canine and feline patients can be challenging. It has been the authors' experience that the BD 4-mL urine culture preservative tube can be employed successfully for culture using a much smaller volume ($\geq$0.5 mL) of urine, when necessary.

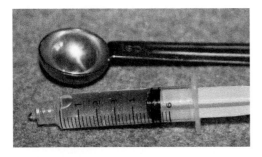

Figure 1.1 The minimum recommended volume for routine urinalysis is 5 mL or 1 teaspoon.

in all patients. Consequently, analysis of post-voided urine collected from a variety of surfaces may be necessary in select cases (Box 1.4 and Figure 1.15). Voided cat urine can sometimes be collected from a clean litter pan to which nonabsorbable plastic beads (e.g. Uri-Void™) or hydrophobic sand (Kit4Cat™) has been added. Cat owners may also use clean glass aquarium beads, straws which have been cut up, or plastic craft beads as litter substitutes. In some cases urine can

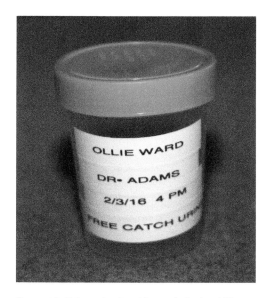

Figure 1.2 Urine submitted for analysis should be submitted in a suitable, capped container with appropriate labeling.

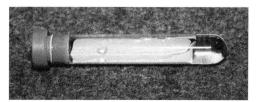

Figure 1.3 Cytologic evaluation of urine can be enhanced by including a urine sample submitted in an EDTA tube.

be successfully collected from a litter pan after a feline patient has voided on top of clinging plastic wrap that has been placed over the cat's usual litter or, in the case of outdoor cats, over a layer of dirt (Figure 1.16). At times the only available urine for analysis is a sample that has been voided onto a floor, tabletop, or other contaminated surface. This contamination factor must be taken into consideration when evaluating such a sample. Prompt examination of the collected urine sample should decrease the level of artifacts encountered. As would be expected, the less contaminated the collection surface, the more reliable the urinalysis results obtained. However, disinfectants used in cleaning the surface from which a urine sample is subsequently obtained also have the potential to alter the urinalysis results, particularly when performing dipstick colorimetric tests. Post-voided urine samples obtained from a surface are generally unsatisfactory for accurate identification of infectious agents, especially if there is a time delay in analysis. At minimum, specific gravity of the urine specimen can usually be determined with reasonable accuracy.

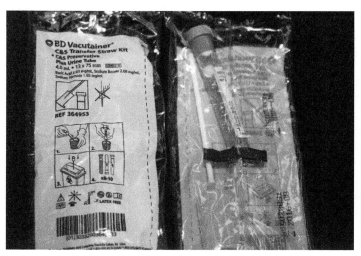

(a)

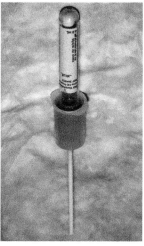

(b)

Figure 1.4 (a) BD Vacutainer® 4-mL urine culture preservative tube kit. (b) Culture preservative tube attached to urine transfer straw.

Box 1.2 Techniques for obtaining free catch urine samples – normal voiding.

Canine Technique

1. If the dog's hair coat around the vulva or prepuce is notably dirty, clean the area and pat dry
2. Walk the dog on a leash early in the morning, after feeding, or at another time that the dog is accustomed to urinating
3. Observe the dog for initiation of micturition and be prepared to collect a sample at the beginning of urination. If desired, latex gloves can be worn by the collector for his/her protection. The collector can plan on positioning the urine container with his/her hands or with a device designed to hold and position the container. Commercial collection devices are available (e.g. Olympic Clean-Catch™) or can be made at home. One such homemade device consists of a yardstick or pole/broom-type handle taped to the handle of a ladle or suitable plastic measuring cup (Figure 1.5). Have one or two suitable containers available for urine collection. The container(s) should be clean and dry and appropriate for the size of the dog. Container(s) may be provided by the veterinarian or a suitable clean, dry household plastic or glass container may be used for urine collection. Smaller dogs may require a flatter collecting receptacle such as a shallow plastic tray, a Styrofoam plate with a raised rim, or a metal, disposable pie plate (Figure 1.6)
4. As soon as micturition is initiated or a micturition posture is assumed, place the collection container as unobtrusively as possible under the vulva, immediately anterior and ventral to the prepuce, or directly in the urine stream produced. If possible, obtain at least 5–10 mL (1–2 tsp) for urinalysis. If the collector is able, a second container (midstream sample) should be positioned for urine collection provided the dog is continuing to urinate after a sample of the initial urine stream has been obtained in the first container (Figure 1.7)
5. The collector should thoroughly wash his/her hands following the collection process
6. After an appropriate urine sample has been obtained, the specimen may need to be transferred to a different, more secure container for transport, depending upon the receptacle used for collection. A lid or plastic wrap cover should be placed over the transport container holding the specimen. In the case where two urine samples have been obtained, an initial stream sample (first container) and a midstream sample (second container), the midstream specimen is the preferred sample for submission. If the urine cannot be taken to a veterinarian or examined within 60 minutes, the sample should be refrigerated unless the collector has been instructed otherwise by the veterinarian. If the specimen was not obtained at the veterinarian's office, the sample should be submitted to the veterinarian as soon as possible

Feline Technique

1. The collector should gradually accustom the cat to being approached and having its hindquarters or tail touched while it is voiding or getting ready to void in the litter box
2. The collector should take note of times when the cat is most likely to urinate to improve his/her opportunity to obtain a urine sample. It is sometimes helpful to restrict the cat's access to the litter box overnight so that the cat will void shortly after regaining access to the box
3. Observe the cat for initiation of micturition in the litter box and have a suitable clean, dry container/device ready to collect urine. The collector may wish to wear latex gloves for his/her protection. The veterinarian may provide a container for urine collection. Usually cats require a flatter container for collection. Often the lid of a veterinarian-provided container will work better for obtaining a sample than the container itself (Figure 1.8). Household containers suitable for feline urine collection include clean, dry, small plastic or glass bowls, small rimmed plates, metal or plastic spoons, or shallow plastic trays – see Figure 1.6

4. As soon as micturition is initiated or a micturition posture is assumed, approach the rear end of the cat and place the collection container as unobtrusively as possible underneath the cat or directly in the urine stream if it can be seen. It may be necessary to gently lift the base of the tail to position the collection receptacle (Figure 1.9). If possible, obtain at least 5–10 mL (1–2 tsp) for urinalysis. Although a midstream sample (urine obtained after initiation of urination and while the cat is producing a steady stream) is preferred for submission, obtaining a true midstream specimen is often difficult to accomplish in the cat

5. The collector should thoroughly wash his/her hands following the collection process

6. After an appropriate urine sample has been obtained, the specimen may need to be transferred to a different, more secure container for transport, depending upon the receptacle used for collection. A lid or plastic wrap cover should be placed over any open transport container holding a specimen. If the urine cannot be taken to a veterinarian or examined within 60 minutes, the sample should be refrigerated unless the collector has been instructed otherwise by the veterinarian. If the specimen was not obtained at the veterinarian's office, the sample should be submitted to the veterinarian as soon as possible

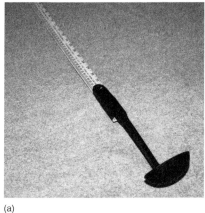 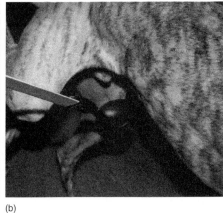

(a)   (b)

Figure 1.5 (a) Homemade urine collection device consisting of a long-handled ladle attached to a yardstick with duct tape. (b) Homemade urine collection device appropriately positioned for collecting urine from a male dog by free-catch method.

Figure 1.6 Common household containers which may be used for free-catch urine collection, depending upon the size of the dog or cat.

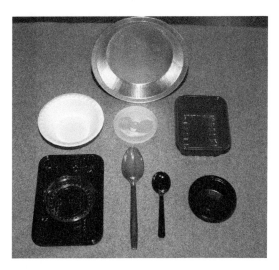

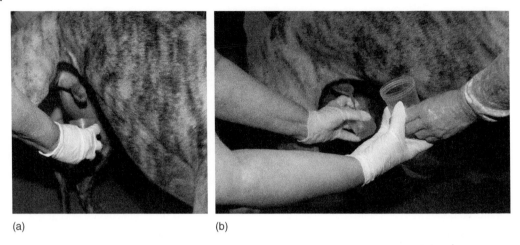

(a)   (b)

Figure 1.7 (a) Appropriate positioning of standard veterinarian-issued urine collection container for a free-catch sample from a male dog. (b) Preparing to hand off a second urine collection container to obtain a mid-stream free-catch sample after an initial micturition sample of 5–10 mL has been obtained.

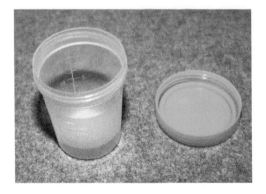

Figure 1.8 Typical veterinarian-issued urine collection container with lid. For cats and small canine patients the container lid often works better for collecting a urine sample during micturition than the container itself.

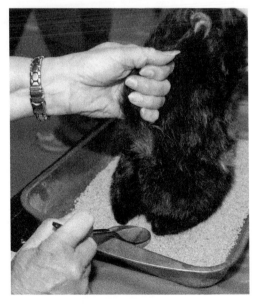

Figure 1.9 Positioning a large spoon or other receptacle posterior and ventral to the hindquarters for free-catch urine collection in the cat may require gently lifting the base of the tail.

Box 1.3 **Techniques for obtaining free-catch urine samples from dogs and cats – manual expression.**

*The manual expression technique for urine collection should **not** be used postoperatively in cystotomy patients and be used with caution in other laparotomy patients. Excessive force should never be used when attempting bladder expression. Initiating a urine stream by manual expression in a male cat can be particularly difficult due to the length and diameter of the urethra, heightening awareness of the potential to produce trauma in the male, feline patient.*

1. If the patient's hair coat around the vulva or prepuce is notably dirty, clean the area and pat dry
2. An assistant may be necessary to help restrain the patient and/or catch the expressed sample depending upon the patient's size, attitude, and health status
3. Have one or two suitable containers available for urine collection:
   a. The container(s) should be clean and dry and appropriate for the size of the patient
   b. Container(s) may be provided by the veterinarian or a suitable clean, dry, household plastic or glass container may be used for urine collection. Smaller dogs and cats may require a flatter collecting receptacle such as a shallow plastic tray, collection container lid, Styrofoam plate with a raised rim, or a metal, disposable pie plate – see Figures 1.6 and 1.8
4. If desired, latex gloves can be worn by the collector for his/her protection
5. For urine collection the patient is most commonly placed in a laterally recumbent or standing position
   a. Dogs or cats in lateral recumbency:
      i. The individual expressing the bladder of a cat or small to medium-sized dog is commonly positioned adjacent to the posterior spine or ventral abdomen or behind the hindquarters of the patient. For a large to giant-sized dog the individual attempting manual compression is usually positioned adjacent to the posterior ventral abdomen. Prior to or during the application of bladder pressure a collection container should be placed immediately posterior to the canine or feline vulva or immediately anterior to the canine prepuce or posterior to the feline prepuce for urine collection, adjusting the container as necessary when urine is expressed
      ii. The bladder can often be palpated as a lemon to orange-sized or larger, fluid-filled structure similar to a water balloon. For cats or small to medium-sized dogs the cupped hand of the individual attempting manual expression should be placed against the patient's ventral abdomen just in front of and, in some cases, slightly under the hind legs. The thumb of the hand should be on one side of the abdomen and the fingers on the other side. The cupped hand should gently push the patient's abdomen up toward the spine while steadily squeezing the walls of the abdomen to produce pressure on the urinary bladder (Figure 1.10). For large to giant-sized dogs the individual attempting bladder expression should place one hand on either side of the caudal abdomen with the fingers of each hand extended toward the spine in front of and slightly under the hindquarters. When both hands are used in bladder expression, the hands should be pressed together gently and steadily to exert pressure on the bladder (Figure 1.11)
   b. Dogs or cats in standing position:
      i. The individual expressing the bladder is generally positioned alongside the body and facing the hindquarters or behind the hindquarters and facing the head. Prior to or during the application of bladder pressure in the dog a urine collection container should be placed immediately posterior and ventral to the vulva or immediately anterior and ventral to the prepuce. For urine collection in the cat the container should be placed immediately posterior to the vulva or prepuce. In both canine and feline patients the position of the container should be adjusted as necessary for collection when urine is expressed

ii. The bladder can often be palpated as a lemon to orange-sized or larger, fluid-filled structure similar to a water balloon. For cats or small to medium-sized dogs, the cupped hand of the individual should be placed against the ventral abdomen in front of or slightly under the hind limbs with the thumb on one side of the abdomen and the fingers on the other side. The cupped hand should gently push the patient's abdomen up toward the spine while steadily squeezing the walls of the abdomen to produce pressure on the urinary bladder (Figure 1.12). When expressing the bladder of a large to giant-sized dog while behind the dog and facing the head, one hand is usually placed on each side of the abdomen with the palm placed below the spine directly in front of the hindquarters and the extended fingers angled downward and cranially. When standing alongside the body of a larger dog while facing the hindquarters, one hand should be placed on each side of the abdomen with the palm positioned below the spine in front of the hindquarters and the extended fingers angled downward and caudally; alternatively, the hands may be placed in a lower position on each side of the abdomen in front of the hindquarters with the extended fingers angled caudally and upward toward the spine (Figure 1.13). Once positioned, the hands should be pressed together gently and steadily to exert pressure on the bladder

c. The two-handed techniques described above for bladder expression of larger dogs may also be used for cats and small to medium-sized dogs. The individual performing manual expression in smaller patients may need only the fingers for application of pressure to the bladder with the palms commonly placed lateral to the spine or below the ventral abdomen

6. Whether the patient is standing or laterally recumbent, if a urine stream has not been produced after 6–10 seconds of appropriate pressure, the hand(s) can be repositioned anteriorly or posteriorly from the original site and pressure reapplied. Because the bladder is a very distensible organ the individual attempting bladder expression may wish to position the hand(s) on the lower abdomen near the thorax and gradually move the hand(s) posteriorly and dorsally as the pelvis is approached; this technique may optimize the chances for bladder palpation and urine expression, especially in larger dogs (Figure 1.14). When a urine stream is produced, the hand or hands should continue to apply pressure inwardly and posteriorly toward the pelvis until a satisfactory specimen is collected (5–10 mL) or only urine dribbling occurs. If the collector is able, a second container (midstream sample) should be positioned for urine collection provided an adequate urine stream is continuing to be expressed following collection of the initial sample

7. Although manual expression attempts do not always produce the desired urine sample, these attempts will sometimes induce the dog or cat to void naturally. Therefore, if manual expression attempts fail to produce a satisfactory urine sample or cause the patient to become too agitated or uncomfortable, the canine patient should be immediately leash-walked or a litter box promptly provided for the feline patient in an attempt to collect a urine sample by natural voiding – see Box 1.2)

8. The collector and person performing manual expression should thoroughly wash their hands following the collection process

9. After an appropriate urine sample has been obtained, the specimen may need to be transferred to a different, more secure container for transport, depending upon the receptacle used for collection. A lid or plastic wrap cover should be placed over any open transport container holding a specimen. In the case where two urine samples have been obtained, an initial stream sample (first container) and a midstream sample (second container), the midstream specimen is the preferred sample for submission. If the urine cannot be taken to a veterinarian or examined within 60 minutes, the sample should be refrigerated unless the collector has been instructed otherwise by the veterinarian. If the specimen was not obtained at the veterinarian's office, the sample should be submitted to the veterinarian as soon as possible

Figure 1.10 Positioning the cupped hand for manual expression of the urinary bladder of the laterally recumbent patient with the hand anterior to the hindquarters, pressing the bladder upward and posteriorly.

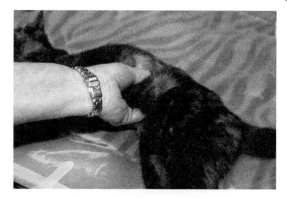

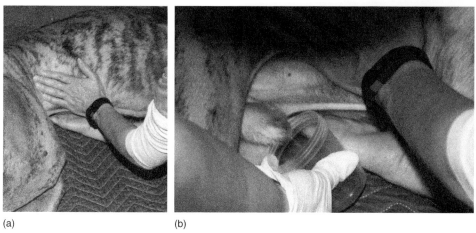

(a)   (b)

Figure 1.11 (a) Demonstration of two-handed manual expression of the urinary bladder of a laterally recumbent dog. Note that the individual performing expression is positioned adjacent to the ventrocaudal abdomen with one hand on either side of the lower abdomen and the fingers extended toward the spine in front of and slightly under the hindquarters. (b) Two-handed manual expression of the urinary bladder of the laterally recumbent dog with the urine collection container appropriately placed anterior to the prepuce of the male patient.

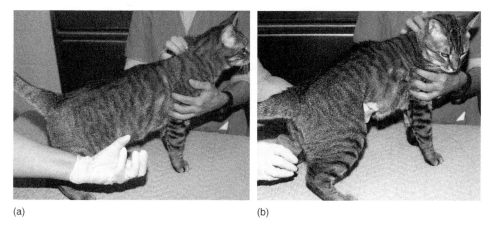

(a)   (b)

Figure 1.12 (a) Demonstration of cupping of hand for manual expression of the urinary bladder of a cat or small to medium-sized dog. (b) Using a cupped hand with the thumb on one side of the patient's abdomen and the fingers on the other side to compress the urinary bladder upward and posteriorly. Note that a collection container is placed appropriately posterior to the hindquarters for catching expressed urine.

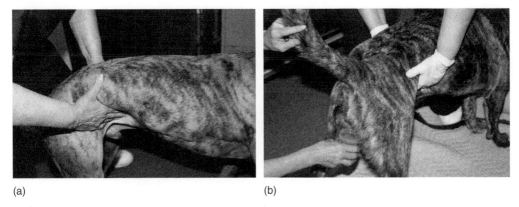

(a)   (b)

Figure 1.13 (a) Demonstration of the two-handed technique for manual expression of the urinary bladder in the dog with the patient standing and the individual performing expression positioned behind the hindquarters and facing the dog's head. Note that one hand is placed on either side of the caudal abdomen with the palm primarily anterior to the hindquarters below the spine and the fingers angled downward and cranially. (b) Demonstration of the two-handed technique for manual expression of the urinary bladder in the dog with the patient standing and the individual performing expression positioned alongside the body of the dog and facing the hindquarters. Note that one hand is placed on each side of the caudal abdomen with the palms positioned below the spine in front of the hindquarters and the extended fingers angled downward and caudally. A urine collection container has been placed appropriately posterior and ventral to the vulva with the patient's tail directed upward to prevent interference with urine collection.

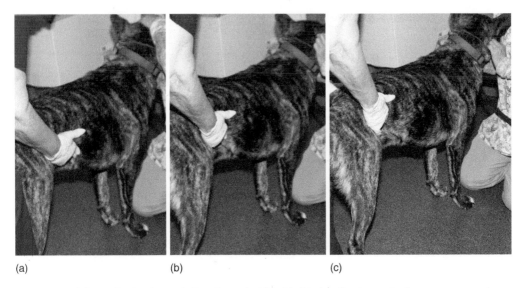

(a)   (b)   (c)

Figure 1.14 Abdominal palpation technique for optimizing bladder localization and subsequent expression, especially in larger patients. Standing behind the dog, the individual attempting to localize the bladder places a hand on either side of the anterior ventral abdomen behind the ribs (a), gently compressing the abdomen inward while gradually moving the hands posteriorly and dorsally (b) until the bladder is palpated or the individual's hands are positioned high in the abdomen in front of the pelvis (c).

Box 1.4 **Techniques for obtaining post-voided urine samples.**

Canine Technique

1. Most post-voided samples obtained in the dog are collected as an unanticipated event, as a planned attempt to obtain a specimen from a dog known to be difficult to collect using other methods, or immediately following unsuccessful attempts to acquire a urine sample through manual expression, transurethral catheterization, or cystocentesis. When planning to obtain post-voided urine or in preparation for voiding that may occur as an inadvertent consequence of attempts to collect urine by other methods, the collector should try to have the dog in a location that has a clean, dry, nonabsorbent surface that will optimize any post-voided sample collection

2. If desired, latex gloves can be worn by the collector for his/her protection

3. When possible, have a suitable device available for aspirating the voided urine such as a clean syringe, pipette, eyedropper, or vacutainer apparatus. These devices can be obtained from the patient's veterinarian or from a commercial source. The minimum amount of urine recommended for collection and submission is 5 mL, although smaller amounts may sometimes be useful, depending on the primary urinalysis objective(s). Collection of post-voided urine, especially when the volume voided is minimal, may be facilitated by consolidating the available urine on the collection surface. Consolidation can be accomplished by placing the straight edge of a microscope slide in contact with the collection surface lengthwise on each side of the available voided urine. One end of each slide should be angled outward so that the two slides form a V-shape. The two slides should be advanced toward each other, causing the urine to run along the bottom of each slide and pooling the urine between them as the end of the slides angled toward the urine come into contact with each other. The pooled urine can then be more easily aspirated or, if the collection surface is elevated such as a table, can be pushed off the edge and caught in a clean container. If microscope slides are unavailable, the clean, straight edges of two stiffly folded pieces of aluminum foil may be used as a substitute (Figure 1.15)

4. The collector should thoroughly wash his/her hands following the collection process

5. After the urine sample has been obtained, the specimen may need to be transferred to a different, more secure container for transport, depending upon the receptacle used for collection. A lid or plastic wrap cover should be placed over any open transport container holding a specimen. The urine submitted should be marked as a post-voided specimen and, ideally, the collection surface should be identified. If the urine cannot be taken to a veterinarian or examined within 60 minutes, the sample should be refrigerated unless the collector has been instructed otherwise by the veterinarian. If the specimen was not obtained at the veterinarian's office, the sample should be submitted to the veterinarian as soon as possible

Feline Technique

1. Most post-voided samples obtained in the cat are collected as a planned attempt to obtain a specimen from a cat known to be difficult to collect using other methods or as a more client- and pet-friendly way of obtaining a specimen. Post-voided sample collection may also be necessary subsequent to an unanticipated voiding event or following voiding precipitated by unsuccessful attempts to acquire a urine sample through manual expression, transurethral catheterization, or cystocentesis. When planning to obtain post-voided urine or in preparation for voiding that may occur as an inadvertent consequence of attempts to collect urine by other methods, the collector should try to have the cat in a location that has a clean, dry, nonabsorbent surface that will optimize any post-voided sample collection. Post-voided urine

collection may be facilitated by providing the feline patient with a commercial pet waste dis-
posal pan with a grate or, more commonly, a typical litter pan that is clean and dry, has litter
covered with plastic wrap clinging to the litter, or has a nonabsorbent litter suitable for urine
collection (see text for additional information about litter pan urine collection)

2. If desired, latex gloves can be worn by the collector for his/her protection
3. When possible, have a suitable device available for aspirating the voided urine such as a clean
syringe, pipette, eyedropper, or vacutainer apparatus. These devices can be obtained from the
patient's veterinarian or from a commercial source. In some cases the voided urine may be
poured into a receptacle directly from the collecting surface. Suitable urine receptacles include
veterinarian-provided containers and common household items such as clean, dry, plastic or
glass containers. The minimum amount of urine recommended for collection and submission
is 5 mL although smaller amounts may sometimes be useful, depending on the primary urinalysis objective(s). Collection of post-voided urine, especially when the volume voided is minimal,
may be facilitated by consolidating the available urine on the collection surface. Consolidation can be accomplished by placing the straight edge of a microscope slide in contact with
the collection surface lengthwise on each side of the available voided urine. One end of each
slide should be angled outward so that the two slides form a V-shape. The two slides should
be advanced toward each other, causing the urine to run along the bottom of each slide and
pooling the urine between them as the end of the slides angled toward the urine come into
contact with each other. The pooled urine can then be more easily aspirated or, if the collection
surface is elevated such as a table, can be pushed off the edge and caught in a clean container.
If microscope slides are unavailable, the clean, straight edges of two stiffly folded pieces of
aluminum foil may be used as a substitute (Figure 1.15)

4. The collector should thoroughly wash his/her hands following the collection process
5. After the urine sample has been obtained, the specimen may need to be transferred to a different, more secure container for transport, depending upon the receptacle used for collection.
A lid or plastic wrap cover should be placed over any open transport container holding a specimen. The urine submitted should be marked as a post-voided specimen and, ideally, the collection surface should be identified. If the urine cannot be taken to a veterinarian or examined
within 60 minutes, the sample should be refrigerated unless the collector has been instructed
otherwise by the veterinarian. If the specimen was not obtained at the veterinarian's office, the
sample should be submitted to the veterinarian as soon as possible

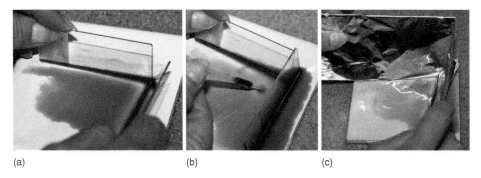

(a)   (b)   (c)

Figure 1.15 Demonstration of technique for consolidation and collection of small amounts of post-voided
urine for analysis. (a) The straight edge of a microscope slide is placed in contact with the collection surface on
each side of the available voided urine and advanced toward each other, forming a V-shape and causing urine
pooling. (b) The consolidated pool allows easier aspiration of urine with a pipette or other instrument. (c) If
microscope slides are unavailable, the clean, straight edges of two stiffly folded pieces of aluminum foil may be
substituted.

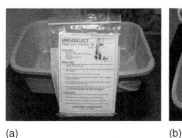 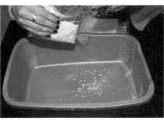 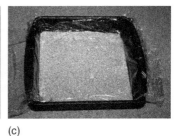

(a) (b) (c)

Figure 1.16 (a) Commercial nonabsorbent beads are available for use in a clean litter pan (b) to assist in collecting voided urine for analysis. (c) Post-voided urine can sometimes be collected from the patient's litter pan by covering the cat's usual litter with clinging plastic wrap.

Transurethral Catheterization

Transurethral catheterization of the urinary bladder is typically performed by trained personnel using a sterile urinary catheter after aseptically cleaning the external genital area and distal urethral opening. Sedation and/or anesthesia may be required for successful catheterization, especially in cats. Advantages with this method are the urinary bladder does not need to be distended to obtain a sample and collection does not depend upon the patient's willingness to urinate. This method does increase the number of red blood cells, transitional cells, and squamous cells present in the urine sample when cells slough off as the catheter passes through the urethra. Catheterization may increase the risk for iatrogenic urinary tract infections (UTIs) as bacteria are introduced into the urinary bladder from the genital tract and distal urethral opening. Patients with hyperadrenocorticism, diabetes mellitus, and renal disease are more at risk for developing UTIs post catheterization. There is risk of both urethral and bladder irritation/trauma and a small risk of perforation for all patients during catheterization. Catheterization may not be possible if there is urethral obstruction.

The risks described for catheterization and potential for alteration of the urine samples obtained by this collection method should limit the use of catheterization to select cases. In addition to adhering to proper technique, the incidence of undesirable sequelae can be diminished through appropriate catheter selection. Ideally, the smallest diameter catheter which is appropriate for the patient should be chosen. Urinary catheters are usually measured in French (Fr) units (1 Fr unit = 0.33 mm) corresponding to the external diameter of the portion of the catheter inserted into the patient's urethra. Suitable catheters for urine collection will vary in diameter depending upon the size of the patient. Typical urinary catheter diameter sizes used in the dog range from 3–10 Fr in both male and female. Typical urinary catheter diameter sizes used in the cat range from 3–5 Fr in male patients and 3–8 Fr in female patients. Urinary catheters will also vary in composition, causing them to fall into flexible, semiflexible, and rigid categories (Figure 1.17). More flexible catheters, especially those composed of silicone, nylon, latex, Teflon, or rubber, will generally create a lesser degree of trauma to the urinary tract and subsequently reduce the number of red blood cells introduced iatrogenically into the urine sample obtained. Some of these more flexible catheters have stylets (Figure 1.18) available to facilitate insertion. Although not as flexible, polypropylene catheters (Figure 1.19) are also commonly used for urine collection. Urinary catheter length ranges from 13 cm (typically used for feline catheterization) to approximately 50 cm (commonly used for canine catheterization). Stainless steel urinary catheters with insertion ends that are angled to facilitate entry into the urethral orifice have sometimes been used for transurethral catheterization of the female dog and cat. Metal catheters usually have a flange attached near the external

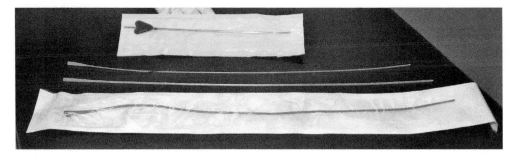

Figure 1.17 Urinary catheters commonly used in male dogs, female dogs and cats. Length and diameter will vary depending upon size of patient. The composition of the catheter also varies, resulting in flexible, semiflexible, and rigid categories of catheters. Pictured top to bottom: stainless steel rigid catheter (female dogs and cats only) – 8 Fr; polypropylene semiflexible catheter – 5 Fr; polypropylene semiflexible catheter – 10 Fr; red rubber flexible catheter – 8 Fr.

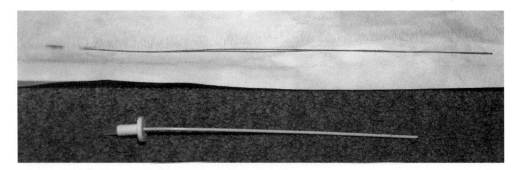

Figure 1.18 Flexible tomcat catheter with appropriate wire stylet.

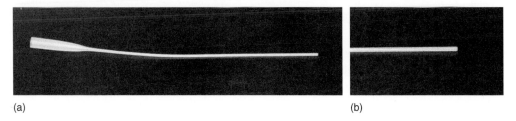

(a)   (b)

Figure 1.19 (a) Standard polypropylene "tomcat" catheter (3.5 Fr, 13 cm) with an open insertion end and a flared external end to prevent catheter migration into the urethra and accommodate syringe attachment. (b) Close-up of catheter open insertion end.

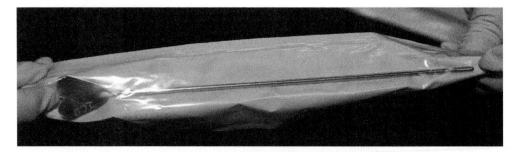

Figure 1.20 Metal female urinary catheter with a flange attached near the external end and a closed-tip insertion end.

Figure 1.21 Example of a urinary catheter (polypropylene) with a closed insertion end with "eye" openings.

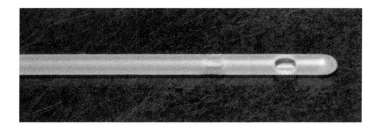

end which helps with both manipulation of the catheter and awareness of the direction in which the insertion end is tipped (Figure 1.20). However, these rigid catheters are not routinely recommended due to the increased likelihood of excessive urethral trauma. Catheters used for urine collection typically have a flared end to prevent migration of the catheter into the urethra and to accommodate a syringe for aspiration. The urethral insertion end of the catheter is commonly tapered and closed. "Eye" openings near the closed end allow urine to enter into the catheter (Figure 1.21). Some catheters do not have eye openings at the insertion end, but are open-ended – see Figure 1.19. Closed-end catheters with eye openings are often preferred for routine urine collection. In the event that the selected catheter does not have a flared end, which is frequently the case for metal catheters, a short segment of flexible tubing can often be used as an adapter to allow the attachment of a syringe (Figure 1.22). Disposable, prepackaged sterile catheters intended for one time use are preferred for patient catheterization rather

than using re-sterilized catheters which may create additional iatrogenic change in the urinalysis results due to products used in the cleaning process.

Although accomplishing transurethral catheterization of the male dog and cat relies on visualization of the urethral orifice (Box 1.5 and Figures 1.23–1.28), there are multiple techniques which can be used to perform transurethral catheterization of the female dog and cat. The technique chosen depends on patient factors such as size, temperament, and vaginal conformation, as well as the experience of the individual performing catheterization. The visualization method for the female of both species uses a speculum and a light source to visualize the urethral papilla and orifice to facilitate catheterization (Box 1.6 and Figures 1.29–1.36). The digital palpation method accomplishes catheterization by use of a finger inserted into the vagina which subsequently directs the tip of the catheter into the urethral orifice (Box 1.7 and Figure 1.37). The digital palpation technique is inappropriate for the cat due to the animal's small size. The blind technique

Figure 1.22 A short segment of a flexible red rubber tube is used here to act as an adapter for the external end of the metal catheter to allow syringe attachment.

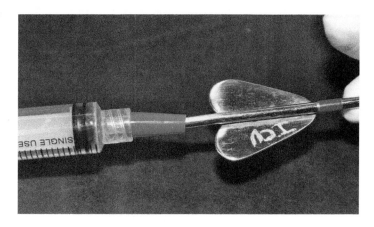

uses neither visualization nor digital palpation but relies on blindly sliding the urinary catheter along the ventral floor of the vagina until it slides through the urethral orifice (Box 1.8 and Figures 1.38, 1.39). The blind technique is most commonly used in smaller patients where visualization or digital palpation methods can be difficult. The digital palpation and blind catheterization techniques put the patient at greater risk for iatrogenic UTIs and urinalysis changes when compared to visualization methods.

Techniques for obtaining canine or feline urine through transurethral catheterization are described in Boxes 1.5, 1.6, 1.7, and 1.8. Transurethral catheterization techniques should always be performed by adequately trained personnel and are **not** recommended for routine use in obtaining urine samples due to the potential risks associated with these techniques. Regardless of the technique chosen, avoiding excessive urogenital trauma should be a primary consideration.

Box 1.5 Male canine and feline transurethral catheterization techniques – visualization method.

Canine Technique

1. Prepare for urine collection:
   a. Have one or two clean/sterile appropriate containers or syringes available for urine collection
   b. Select a suitable sterile urinary catheter appropriate in composition, diameter, and length for the patient (see text for guidelines). The adequacy of catheter length can be checked by holding the catheter lateral to the patient with the flared end just cranial to the prepuce/penis and approximating the urethral pathway by following the length of the catheter as it is extended toward the hind end of the patient. As the hind end of the patient is reached, the catheter should be curved upward and then cranially in the area of the pelvis to approximate the curvature of the urethra as it traverses the ischial arch prior to entering the bladder. If, after following the ischial arch, the insertion end of the catheter will extend anterior to the hindquarters, the catheter should be of sufficient length to reach the bladder. Care should be taken to keep the catheter to be used for urine collection sterile by approximating length while the catheter remains in the sterile packaging or wearing sterile gloves when handling a catheter that has been removed from its wrap and held adjacent to the patient for catheter length evaluation (Figure 1.23)
   c. Sedate the patient, if needed, due to patient temperament or pain (sedation is generally unnecessary for the majority of canine patients)
2. Male dogs are typically positioned in lateral recumbency by an assistant, but larger patients are sometimes catheterized while in a standing position. After positioning the patient, the assistant should retract the prepuce and expose the distal portion of the penis by using one hand to gently push the dorsal aspect of the prepuce at its juncture with the ventral abdomen caudally while using the other hand to grasp the penis through the prepuce, pushing the penis and urethral orifice forward cranial to the prepuce (Figures 1.24, 1.25). Ideally, the urethral orifice of the penis should remain exposed until the catheterization process has been completed
3. The distal end of the prepuce and exposed penis should be gently cleaned with water, sterile sponges, and a disinfecting soap such as chlorhexidine, and then thoroughly rinsed to prevent both infection and iatrogenic changes in urinalysis results. Longer hair that may interfere with or contaminate the catheterization process may be clipped, if necessary
4. Wearing sterile gloves, the person performing catheterization should apply sterile lubricant to the insertion end of the catheter and place it into the urethral orifice. The catheter is then slowly and steadily advanced, remembering that resistance will be met during passage, especially at

the level of the base of the os penis and at the ischial arch. Resistance to catheter passage may sometimes be overcome by gentle rotation of the catheter while pushing it forward. The catheter should be advanced until just past the point where urine starts dripping from the end of the catheter or until the catheter has been inserted to the point where it starts to flare. If the selected catheter meets severe resistance, consideration should be given to attempting passage of a urinary catheter which is smaller in diameter. As an alternative approach to catheterization, the end of the package containing the sterile catheter can be cut open and a section of the packaging can be cut off and freed from the remainder of the catheter sleeve; subsequently, the insertion end of the catheter can be exposed and lubricated, using the freed section of the catheter packaging to handle the catheter in a sterile manner while advancing it through the urethral orifice and on into the bladder lumen. Sterile gloves are not required for the alternative method of catheterization (Figure 1.26). Ideally, the final placement of the catheter tip should be no more than a few centimeters cranial to the neck of the bladder, avoiding over-insertion. Over-insertion can cause bladder trauma, make urine collection more difficult, and/or cause the catheter tip to wrap around the bladder lining and retroflex back through the bladder neck. Discontinuing further catheter advancement after 1–2 cm past the point at which urine first begins to flow from the external end of the catheter will help avoid over-insertion

5. Ideally, a 5–10-mL sample of urine should be collected for submission by catching urine flowing freely out of the catheter into a suitable container or by aspirating the desired amount through a syringe attached to the flared catheter end. If urine is flowing freely or can be aspirated after obtaining the initial sample, a second sample should be collected into a different container or syringe. If obtained, the second urine sample is the preferred sample for submission and analysis or culture since it has a lesser chance of contamination or collection artifact

6. Following completion of urine collection, the urinary catheter should be gently removed by steadily withdrawing the catheter from the urogenital tract in a sterile manner

Feline Technique

1. Prepare for urine collection:
   a. Have one or two clean/sterile appropriate containers or syringes available for urine collection
   b. Select a suitable sterile urinary catheter appropriate in composition, diameter, and length for the patient (see text for guidelines). Although the catheter should be of sufficient length to reach the bladder, the relatively short length of the urethra in the male cat generally permits transurethral catheterization using a standard "tomcat" catheter (3.5 Fr, 13 cm) – see Figure 1.19a. Longer catheters can be used but are usually not needed for short-term feline catheterization. If a longer catheter is used, care should be taken to prevent over-insertion so that complications, such as bladder trauma, urine collection impairment, and catheter retroflexion into the urethra, do not occur. Although the diameter of the feline urethra may accommodate a larger catheter than the 3.5 Fr size often chosen for short-term use, catheterization with larger-diameter catheters increases the possibility of excessive urethral trauma
   c. Sedation of the male feline patient is often required for humane, successful transurethral catheterization
   d. Sterile gloves should be worn when performing transurethral catheterization

2. Male cats are typically positioned in lateral recumbency when sedated. Using an assistant or mechanical restraint such as ties or adhesive wrap, the hind limbs should ideally be extended cranially and the tail dorsally and cranially to optimize exposure of the prepuce (Figure 1.27). When catheterization is performed in the awake patient, positioning may vary depending upon the condition of the cat, but optimizing preputial exposure should still be a primary objective

3. The prepuce and adjacent tissue should be cleaned with sterile sponges, water, and a disinfecting soap such as chlorhexidine, and then thoroughly rinsed to prevent both infection and iatrogenic changes in the urinalysis results. Longer hair that may interfere with or contaminate the catheterization process may be clipped, if necessary (Figure 1.27)

4. Wearing sterile gloves, the person performing catheterization should apply sterile lubricant to the insertion end of the selected catheter. Using one gloved hand, the penis should be exposed by pushing the prepuce back against the body. With the other gloved hand, the lubricated catheter tip is inserted into the urethral orifice. With the fingers gently compressing the penis against the inserted catheter, the penis should be extended away from the body posteriorly and approximately parallel to the long axis of the body to facilitate further catheter insertion (Figure 1.28). The catheter should then be gently but firmly pushed retrograde through the urethra and into the bladder until urine is dripping freely from the flared end or the catheter has been fully inserted up to the flared end (or a length approximating the 13-cm length of a typical "tomcat" catheter if using a catheter of longer length). Excessive force should be avoided in order to prevent urethral trauma and iatrogenic urine artifact. Over-insertion of longer catheters can be avoided by discontinuing catheter advancement 1–2 cm after the point at which urine flow is initially observed

5. Ideally, a 5–10-mL sample of urine should be collected for submission by catching urine flowing freely out of the catheter into a suitable container or by aspirating the desired amount into a syringe attached to the flared catheter end. If urine is flowing freely or can be aspirated after obtaining the initial sample, a second sample should be collected into a different container or syringe. If obtained, the second urine sample is the preferred sample for submission and analysis or culture since it has a lesser chance of contamination or collection artifact

6. Following completion of urine collection, the urinary catheter should be gently removed from the urogenital tract by steady withdrawal in a sterile manner

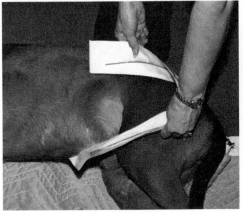 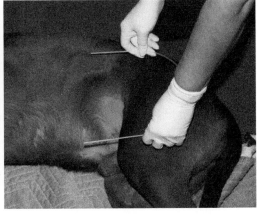

(a) (b)

Figure 1.23 Demonstration of determining adequacy of urinary catheter length in the male dog without (a) and with (b) sterile gloves by holding the catheter adjacent to the lateral aspect of the patient's body and approximating the course of the urethra from the urethral orifice to the neck of the bladder. Catheter length is judged to be sufficient if the insertion end extends anterior to the hindquarters when the flared end is held just cranial to the prepuce/penis and the curve around the ischial arch has been approximated.

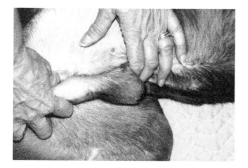 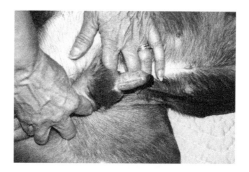

Figure 1.24 Demonstration of canine penis and urethral orifice exposure for urinary catheterization. An assistant can expose the penis/urethral orifice by using one hand to gently push the dorsal aspect of the prepuce caudally.

Figure 1.25 Urethral orifice exposure is enhanced by the assistant continuing to push the dorsal aspect of the prepuce caudally while using the other hand to grasp the penis through the prepuce and push it forward cranial to the prepuce. (The patient pictured has an incidental urethral prolapse.)

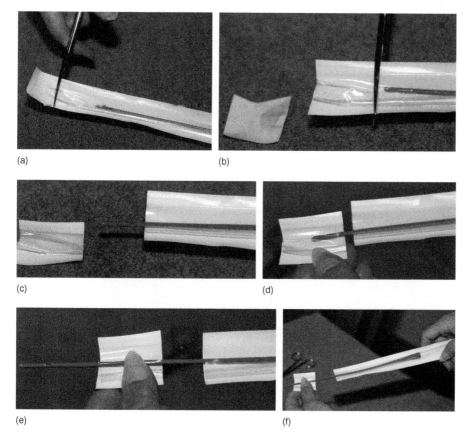

Figure 1.26 Demonstration of urinary catheter handling technique in which a sterile segment of catheter packaging can be used to handle the catheter, eliminating the need for sterile gloves. (a) The end of the catheter packaging is cut off to open the catheter sleeve. (b) A second segment of the catheter packaging is cut and separated from the sterile insertion end of the catheter still in the sleeve. (c) The sterile insertion end is pushed out of the open sleeve. (d) The sterile insertion end is inserted through the freed segment of sterile packaging without directly touching the exposed sterile catheter. (e) The freed packaging segment can now be used to handle the urinary catheter, keeping it sterile for lubrication of the insertion end and subsequent introduction into the urethra. (f) The remainder of the catheter can be gradually pulled out of the sterile sleeve and pushed progressively into the urethra, using the freed packaging segment.

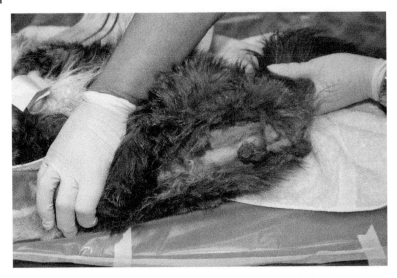

Figure 1.27 Preparation for transurethral catheterization of the male feline patient. The cat has been sedated, placed in lateral recumbency, and the genital area has been scrubbed and clipped (clipping is optional). Note that the hind limbs have been pulled cranially and the tail has been pulled dorsally and cranially to optimize exposure of the prepuce.

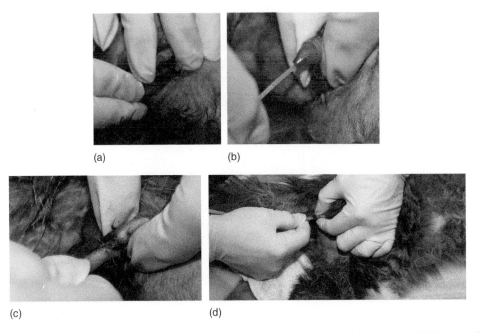

Figure 1.28 Demonstration of initial steps in transurethral catheterization of the male cat. (a) Using sterile gloves, the prepuce of the sedated and prepped patient is pushed back against the body to expose the penis. (b) The lubricated insertion end of the sterile urinary catheter is inserted into the urethral orifice. (c, d) The penis is gently compressed around the catheter, extending the penis away from the body dorsally and approximately parallel to the long axis of the body in order to facilitate further catheter insertion.

Box 1.6 Female canine and feline transurethral catheterization techniques – visualization method.

Canine Technique

1. Prepare for urine collection:
   a. Have one or two clean/sterile appropriate containers or syringes available for urine collection
   b. Select a suitable sterile urinary catheter appropriate in composition, diameter, and length for the patient (see text for guidelines). Sterile red rubber or other catheters of flexible materials and polypropylene catheters are frequently used in the transurethral catheterization of female dogs. Although care should be taken to choose a catheter of sufficient length to reach the bladder, most catheters standardly used for catheterization of female dogs are several centimeters in length and capable of reaching the bladder. If uncertain that the catheter length is sufficient, the catheter in its sterile packaging, or held with sterile gloves when out of its wrapper, can be placed lateral to the hind end of the patient with the flared end just caudal to the vulva and the remainder of the catheter approximating the urethral pathway upward and then cranially to the bladder. If the insertion end of the catheter extends anterior to the hindquarters, catheter length should be sufficient to reach the bladder (Figure 1.29)
   c. If anticipating the use of a stylet with a flexible catheter, select a sterile stylet appropriate for the catheter chosen. Sterile lubricant should be lightly applied to the end of the stylet prior to its insertion into the catheter in order to facilitate withdrawal of the stylet when appropriate (Figure 1.30)
   d. A sterile speculum suitable for the patient and an external light source should be provided. An otoscope consisting of a handle, a head with an attached light source and a movable lens, and appropriately sized cones for attachment can be used (Figure 1.31). Larger otoscope cones will allow better visualization, but size of the patient, diameter of the selected urinary catheter, and vulvar conformation can be limiting factors. Stainless steel human nasal speculums can also be used (author prefers Killian nasal speculum with 2–3.5-inch [5–9-cm] blades depending upon patient size), but require a light source such as an adjustable, free-standing light, an assistant-held penlight or transilluminator, or a head lamp (Figure 1.32)
   e. Sedate the patient, if needed, due to patient temperament or pain (sedation is generally unnecessary for the majority of canine patients)
   f. Sterile gloves should be worn when performing this method of transurethral catheterization
2. An assistant will be needed to restrain the nonsedated female patient in a standing (most common position for nonsedated patient) or ventrally recumbent position. Dogs with longer tails will need to have the tail directed away from the vulva by the assistant or using ties or adhesive wrap. Patients in ventral recumbency should have the hind legs positioned so that the limbs are not interfering with the catheterization process
3. The vulva and adjacent skin should be cleaned with water, sterile sponges, and a disinfecting soap such as chlorhexidine, and then thoroughly rinsed to prevent both infection and iatrogenic changes in urinalysis results. Longer hair that may interfere with or contaminate the catheterization process may be clipped, if necessary
4. Wearing sterile gloves, the person performing catheterization should apply sterile lubricant to the outside of the insertion end of the sterile cone that has been attached to the otoscope with the light source on. The assembled otoscope can be held with a sterile wrap or the hand holding the otoscope can be considered nonsterile and subsequently not be allowed to contact sterile surfaces or equipment. The lubricated cone is inserted gently through the vulva, sliding it along the dorsal wall of the vestibule until past the clitoral fossa. The cone should then be directed cranially and ventrally toward the vagina. Observing through the lens of the otoscope,

the individual catheterizing the patient should be able to see the urethral orifice in the urethral papilla come into view as the floor of the pelvis is approached. After the urethral orifice is visualized, the lubricated insertion end of the selected catheter should be passed by the sterile-gloved hand through the otoscope cone, urethral orifice, and urethra into the bladder lumen (Figure 1.33). Over-insertion of the catheter should be avoided by discontinuing advancement of the catheter 1–2 cm after the point at which urine flow is initially observed. If a stylet has been used to assist in the catheterization process, it should be withdrawn from the catheter lumen. The otoscope handle with head can be detached from the cone and set aside. However, the flared end of the inserted catheter will generally not allow the otoscope cone to be completely separated from the catheter inserted through it until the catheter is withdrawn following urine collection. Alternatively, a sterile, stainless steel human nasal speculum appropriate for the size of the patient may be used in conjunction with a separate external light source to accomplish visual transurethral catheterization. After sterile lubricant is applied to the blades of the nasal speculum, the individual performing catheterization uses his/her gloved hand to hold the handle of the speculum in an upward direction with the blades positioned below. The lubricated blades are then passed in a closed position through the vulva, gently sliding the blades dorsally along the vestibule wall to avoid the clitoral fossa. Once the blades have been introduced as far as possible dorsally and meet resistance, they are then directed cranially and ventrally until the blades are well inserted into or near the vagina in a position parallel to the long axis of the dog. Once insertion is completed, the blades of the speculum are opened gently, and the external light source is positioned so that the urethral orifice can be observed. After the urethral orifice is visualized, the lubricated insertion end of the selected catheter is passed by a sterile-gloved hand through the urethral orifice and urethra into the bladder lumen. Over-insertion of the catheter should be avoided. If a stylet has been used to assist in the catheterization process, it should be withdrawn from the catheter lumen. When urine appears in the catheter by free flow or aspiration with a syringe, the speculum blades may be left in place until a sample is obtained or gently withdrawn from the genital tract, being careful not to dislodge the catheter from the bladder lumen (Figure 1.34)

5. Ideally, a 5–10-mL sample of urine should be collected for submission by catching urine flowing freely out of the catheter into a suitable container or by aspirating the desired amount into a syringe attached to the flared catheter end. If urine is flowing freely or can be aspirated after obtaining the initial sample, a second sample should be collected into a different container or syringe. If obtained, the second urine sample is the preferred sample for submission and analysis or culture since it has a lesser chance of contamination or collection artifact
6. Following completion of urine collection, the urinary catheter and speculum, if still present, should be gently removed from the urogenital tract by steady withdrawal in a sterile manner

Feline Technique

1. Prepare for urine collection:
   a. Have one or two clean/sterile appropriate containers or syringes available for urine collection
   b. Select a suitable sterile urinary catheter appropriate in composition, size, and length for the patient (see text for guidelines). Although the catheter should be of sufficient length to reach the bladder, the relatively short length of the urethra in the female cat generally permits transurethral catheterization using a standard "tomcat" catheter (approximately 3.5 Fr, 13 cm); see Figure 1.19a. Longer catheters can be used but are usually not needed for short-term feline catheterization. If a longer catheter is used, care should be taken to prevent over-insertion so that complications, such as bladder trauma, urine collection impairment,

and catheter retroflexion into the urethra, do not occur. Although the diameter of the feline urethra may accommodate a larger catheter than the 3.5 Fr size often chosen for short-term use, catheters larger in diameter can potentially produce more trauma to the urethra

   c. If anticipating the use of a stylet with a flexible catheter, select a sterile stylet appropriate for the catheter chosen (see Figure 1.18). Sterile lubricant should be lightly applied to the end of the stylet prior to its insertion into the catheter in order to facilitate withdrawal of the stylet when appropriate (see Figure 1.30)

   d. A sterile speculum, suitable for the patient, and an external light source should be provided. An otoscope consisting of a handle, a head with an attached light and a movable lens, and appropriately sized cones for attachment can be used (Figure 1.35). A larger cone will allow better visualization, but the small size of most feline patients limits both the size of the speculum and the size of the catheter that can be passed through an otoscope cone

   e. Sedation of the female feline patient is usually required for humane, successful transurethral catheterization

   f. Sterile gloves should be worn when performing this method of transurethral catheterization

2. Sedated female cats are often positioned in ventral recumbency. Using an assistant or mechanical restraint such as ties or an adhesive wrap, the tail should be positioned away from the area of the vulva. The hind limbs should be positioned in a flexed position alongside the body or, assuming the patient is sufficiently sedated and has been placed on an elevated surface, can be allowed to hang downward from the table top

3. The vulva and adjacent skin should be cleaned with water, sterile sponges, and a disinfecting soap such as chlorhexidine, and then thoroughly rinsed to prevent both infection and iatrogenic changes in urinalysis results. Longer hair that may interfere with or contaminate the catheterization process may be clipped, if necessary

4. Wearing sterile gloves, the person performing catheterization should apply sterile lubricant to the outside of the insertion end of the sterile cone that has been attached to the otoscope with the light source on. The otoscope handle can be held with a sterile wrap or the hand holding the otoscope can be considered nonsterile and subsequently not be allowed to contact sterile surfaces or equipment. The lubricated speculum is inserted gently through the vulva, sliding it along the dorsal wall of the vestibule until past the clitoral fossa. Observing through the lens of the otoscope, the individual catheterizing the patient should be able to see the urethral orifice in the urethral papilla come into view as the floor of the pelvis is approached (Figure 1.36). After the urethral orifice is visualized, the lubricated insertion end of the selected catheter is passed by the sterile-gloved hand through the otoscope cone, urethral orifice, and urethra into the bladder lumen. Discontinuing catheter advancement 1–2 cm after the point at which initial urine flow from the catheter has been observed will help avoid over-insertion of the catheter. If a stylet has been used to assist in the catheterization process, it should be withdrawn from the catheter lumen. The otoscope handle with head can be detached from the cone and set aside. However, the flared end of the inserted catheter will generally not allow the otoscope cone to be completely separated from the catheter inserted through it until the catheter is withdrawn following urine collection

5. Ideally, a 5–10-mL sample of urine should be collected for submission by catching urine flowing freely out of the catheter into a suitable container or by aspirating the desired amount into a syringe attached to the flared catheter end. If urine is flowing freely or can be aspirated after obtaining the initial sample, a second sample should be collected into a different container or syringe. If obtained, the second urine sample is the preferred sample for submission and analysis or culture since it has a lesser chance of contamination or collection artifact

6. Following completion of urine collection, the urinary catheter and otoscope cone should be gently removed from the urogenital tract by steady withdrawal in a sterile manner

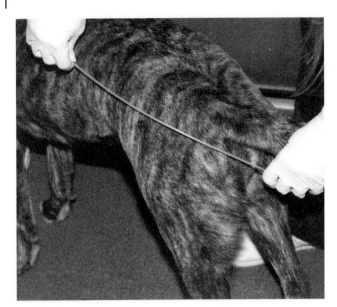

Figure 1.29 When uncertain if the length of the urinary catheter chosen is sufficient to reach the urinary bladder in the female dog, the catheter can be held lateral to the body of the dog, holding the flared end caudal to the vulva and approximating the course of the urethra upward from the vagina and then cranially to the neck of the bladder. The length should be sufficient if the insertion end of the catheter extends anterior to the hindquarters of the patient. Sterile gloves should be worn and care taken not to contaminate the catheter if the catheter is not wrapped in sterile packaging when the length is evaluated.

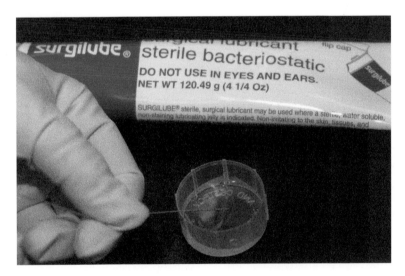

Figure 1.30 If a urinary catheter stylet is used in the transurethral catheterization process, sterile lubricant should be lightly applied to the end of the stylet prior to its insertion into the catheter in order to facilitate withdrawal of the stylet when appropriate.

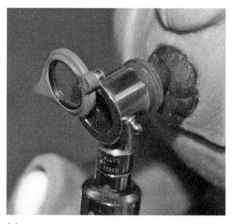

(a)

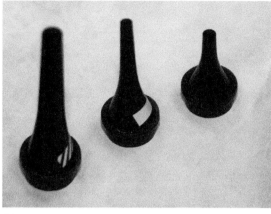

(b)

Figure 1.31 (a) Otoscope with handle, head with attached light source and movable lens, and fitted with a cone speculum suitable for transurethral catheterization of the female patient by the visualization method. (b) Varying otoscope cone sizes which can be used for visualization of the female canine urethral orifice in transurethral catheterization.

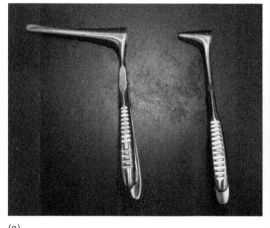

(a)

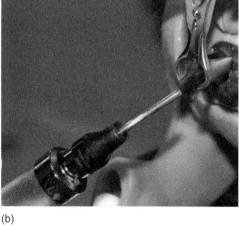

(b)

Figure 1.32 (a) Stainless steel nasal speculums for humans which can be used for female canine transurethral catheterization by the visualization method. (b) A transilluminator is one possible light source which can be used for visualization when using a stainless steel nasal speculum for transurethral catheterization.

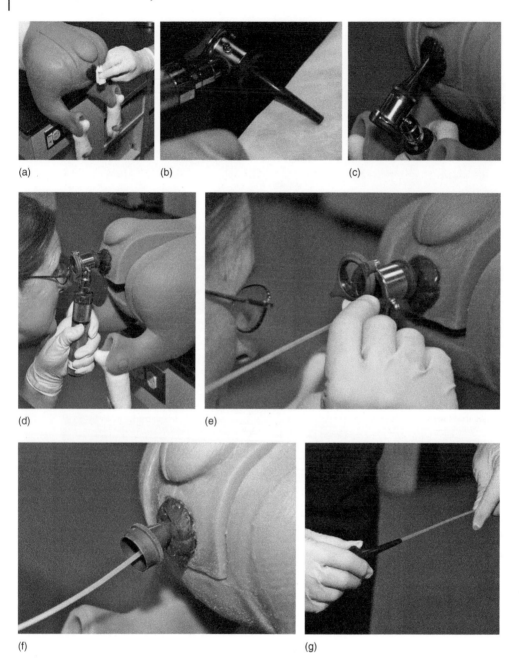

Figure 1.33 Demonstration of transurethral catheterization by visualization of the urethral orifice with an otoscope using a female canine catheterization mannequin positioned in ventral recumbency. (a) The vaginal area has been cleansed. (b) Sterile lubricant is applied to the narrow end of the sterile cone attached to the otoscope. (c) The otoscope cone is inserted through the vulva and upward along the dorsal wall of the vestibule until past the area of the clitoral fossa. (d) The individual performing the procedure then directs the cone cranially and slightly ventrally until the urethral orifice comes into view. (e) After pushing the otoscope lens partially to the side, the selected lubricated catheter is passed in a sterile manner through the cone, urethral orifice, and urethra into the urinary bladder. (f) After catheter entry into the bladder, the otoscope head and handle can be detached from the cone and set aside. (g) The cone can be removed from the genital tract, but generally not completely separated from the catheter until catheter removal subsequent to urine collection.

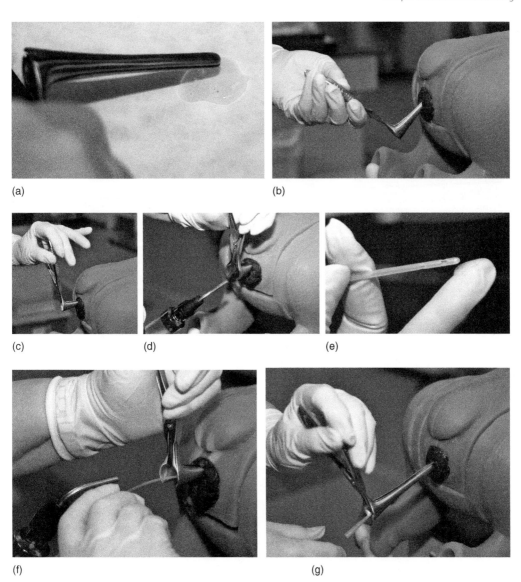

Figure 1.34 Demonstration of transurethral catheterization by visualization of the urethral orifice with a nasal speculum and external light source using a female canine catheterization mannequin positioned in ventral recumbency. (a) Wearing sterile gloves, the individual performing catheterization applies sterile lubricant to the blades of the selected nasal speculum. (b) Holding the handle of the speculum in an upward direction with the blades below in a closed position, the speculum blades are inserted into the vulva in an upward direction in order to traverse the vestibule dorsally. (c) After passing through the vestibule dorsally, the blades are directed cranially and slightly ventrally until they are well inserted into the vagina. (d) The blades are then gently opened and a transilluminator or other external light source is used to locate the urethral orifice. (e) Sterile lubricant is applied to the insertion end of the selected catheter. (f) The catheter is then passed by a sterile-gloved hand between the blades and through the urethral orifice and urethra into the urinary bladder. (g) After the catheter is placed into the bladder, the speculum blades can be left in place until a urine sample is obtained, or can be removed from the genital tract, being careful not to dislodge the catheter.

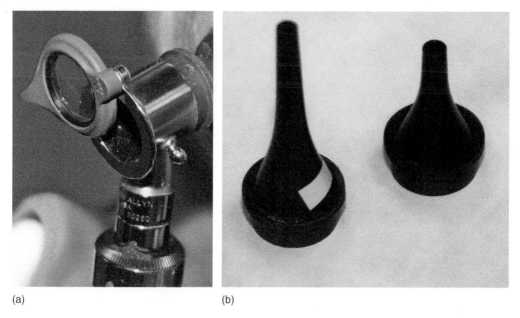

(a)   (b)

Figure 1.35 (a) An otoscope with a handle and a head with an attached light and movable lens is suitable for transurethral catheterization by the visualization method in the female cat. (b) Cone speculums suitable for otoscope attachment and visualization of the urethral orifice of cats.

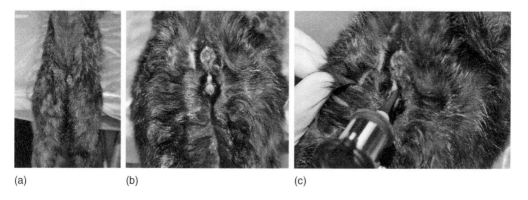

(a)   (b)   (c)

Figure 1.36 Use of otoscopic speculum for transurethral catheterization in the female cat. (a) Sedated female cat in ventral recumbency with limbs hanging down from table top and tail directed upward away from vulva. (b) Cleansed vulva and perivulvar area. (c) Small, sterilized cone attached to otoscope head and handle. The lubricated insertion end of the cone is inserted through the vulva approximately parallel to the long axis of the cat's body, sliding it along the dorsal vestibule wall and into the vagina until the urethral orifice is visualized. A small-diameter, lubricated catheter can then be sterilely introduced through the cone, urethral orifice, and urethra into the urinary bladder for urine collection.

Box 1.7 Female canine transurethral catheterization technique – digital palpation method.

1. Prepare for urine collection:
   a. Have one or two clean/sterile appropriate containers or syringes available for urine collection
   b. Select a suitable sterile urinary catheter appropriate in composition, diameter, and length for the patient (see text for guidelines). Sterile red rubber or other catheters of flexible materials and polypropylene catheters are frequently used in the transurethral catheterization of female dogs. Although care should be taken to choose a catheter of sufficient length to reach the bladder, most catheters standardly used for catheterization of female dogs are several centimeters in length and capable of reaching the bladder. If uncertain that the catheter length is sufficient, the catheter, in its sterile packaging or held by sterile gloves when out of its wrapper, can be placed lateral to the hind end of the patient with the flared end just caudal to the vulva and the remainder of the catheter approximating the urethral pathway upward and then cranially to the bladder. If the insertion end of the catheter extends anterior to the hindquarters, catheter length should be sufficient to reach the bladder (see Figure 1.29)
   c. If anticipating the use of a stylet with a flexible catheter, select a sterile stylet appropriate for the catheter chosen. Sterile lubricant should be lightly applied to the end of the stylet prior to its insertion into the catheter in order to facilitate withdrawal of the stylet when appropriate (see Figure 1.30)
   d. Sedate the patient, if necessary due to patient temperament or pain (sedation is generally unnecessary for the majority of canine patients)
   e. Sterile gloves should be worn when performing this method of transurethral catheterization
2. An assistant will be needed to restrain the nonsedated female patient in a standing (most common position for nonsedated patient) or ventrally recumbent position. Dogs with longer tails will need to have the tail directed away from the vulva by the assistant or through ties or adhesive wrap. Patients in ventral recumbency should have the hind legs positioned so that the limbs are not interfering with the catheterization process
3. The vulva and adjacent skin should be cleaned with water, sterile sponges, and a disinfecting soap such as chlorhexidine, and then thoroughly rinsed to prevent both infection and iatrogenic changes in urinalysis results. Longer hair that may interfere with or contaminate the catheterization process may be clipped, if necessary
4. Depending on the size of the dog and the finger size of the individual performing catheterization, a finger on one hand is selected to perform digital palpation. After gloving, sterile lubricant is applied to the selected finger, which is then inserted through the vulva and advanced along the wall of the vestibule dorsally and then cranially into the vagina until the tip of the finger can be rested on the floor of the pelvis. The other gloved hand is used to insert the lubricated insertion end of the catheter through the vulva into the vestibule and vagina, sliding it underneath the finger resting on the pelvic floor. The catheter end is pushed cranially until it can be felt to slip into the urethral orifice. The urethral papilla and orifice often cannot be distinguished by initial palpation, but upon entry into the orifice, the catheter will push up mucosa dorsally against the fingertip as it is advanced into the urethra. If the catheter continues to be advanced cranially, but only the catheter is felt underneath the finger rather than mucosa overlying the dorsal urethra, then it is probable that the catheter has bypassed the urethra and is being advanced vaginally. If it is suspected that the catheter has bypassed the urethral orifice, the catheter should be withdrawn and re-directed by the finger inserted into the vagina until the urethral orifice can be identified as previously described or it is determined that another

method of urine collection is necessary. Excessive trauma should be avoided in the catheterization process. After the insertion end of the catheter has entered the urethral orifice, the catheter should be steadily and gently advanced until urine flows freely from the catheter or urine can be aspirated into the catheter by a syringe. Over-insertion should be avoided. The finger used to direct the catheter into the urethral orifice can be withdrawn from the urogenital tract after the catheter has entered the urethral orifice or bladder lumen (Figure 1.37). If a stylet has been used in the catheterization process, it should be removed prior to any urine aspiration attempts

5. Ideally, a 5–10-mL sample of urine should be collected for submission by catching urine flowing freely out of the catheter into a suitable container or by aspirating the desired amount into a syringe attached to the flared catheter end. If urine is flowing freely or can be aspirated after obtaining the initial sample, a second sample should be collected into a different container or syringe. If obtained, the second urine sample is the preferred sample for submission and analysis or culture since it has a lesser chance of contamination or collection artifact

6. Following completion of urine collection, the urinary catheter should be gently removed from the urogenital tract by steady withdrawal in a sterile manner

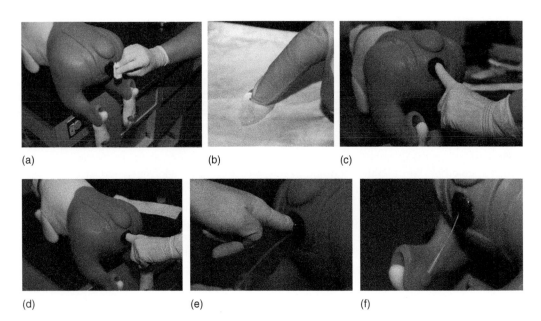

(a) (b) (c)

(d) (e) (f)

Figure 1.37 Demonstration of transurethral catheterization of the female dog by the digital palpation method using a canine female catheterization mannequin positioned in ventral recumbency. (a) The vaginal area is cleansed. (b) Sterile lubricant is applied to the sterile glove covering the finger selected for digital palpation. (c) The finger is then inserted through the vulva in an upward direction, sliding along the dorsal wall of the vestibule. (d) The finger is then moved cranially and slightly ventrally until the it rests on the pelvic floor. (e) Using the other gloved hand, the lubricated insertion end of the selected urinary catheter is inserted through the vulva and underneath the finger resting on the pelvic floor. As the catheter tip is pushed further cranially, the inserted finger helps direct the catheter into the urethral orifice. (f) When catheterization of the urinary bladder has been accomplished, the inserted finger can be withdrawn from the genital tract, being careful not to dislodge the catheter, and the catheter can then be used for urine collection.

Box 1.8 Female canine and feline transurethral catheterization techniques – blind method.

Canine Technique

1. Prepare for urine collection:
   a. Have one or two clean/sterile appropriate containers or syringes available for urine collection
   b. Select a suitable sterile urinary catheter appropriate in composition, diameter, and length for the patient (see text for guidelines). Sterile red rubber or other catheters of flexible materials and polypropylene catheters are frequently used in the transurethral catheterization of female dogs. When more flexible catheters are used for the blind technique, it is often helpful to employ a stylet, giving added stiffness to the catheter in an attempt to facilitate tip insertion into the urethral orifice. Stainless steel catheters with angled insertion tips can also be advantageous in facilitating blind insertion, but must be used with the utmost care because of increased potential for urogenital trauma (see Figure 1.17). Although care should be taken to choose a catheter of sufficient length to reach the bladder, most catheters standardly used for catheterization of female dogs are several centimeters in length and capable of reaching the bladder. If uncertain that the catheter length is sufficient, the catheter, in its sterile packaging or held with sterile gloves without its wrapper, can usually be placed lateral to the hind end of the patient with the flared end just caudal to the vulva and the remainder of the catheter approximating the urethral pathway upward and then cranially to the bladder. If the insertion end of the catheter extends anterior to the hindquarters, catheter length should be sufficient to reach the bladder (see Figure 1.29)
   c. Sedate the patient, if necessary, due to patient temperament or pain (sedation is generally unnecessary for the majority of canine patients)
   d. Sterile gloves should be worn when performing this method of transurethral catheterization
2. An assistant will be needed to restrain the nonsedated female patient in a standing (most common position for nonsedated patient) or ventrally recumbent position. Dogs with longer tails will need to have the tail directed away from the vulva by the assistant or through ties or adhesive wrap. Patients in ventral recumbency should have the hind legs positioned so that the limbs are not interfering with the catheterization process
3. The vulva and adjacent skin should be cleaned with water, sterile sponges, and a disinfecting soap such as chlorhexidine, and then thoroughly rinsed to prevent both infection and iatrogenic changes in urinalysis results. Longer hair that may interfere with or contaminate the catheterization process may be clipped, if necessary
4. Wearing sterile gloves, the person performing catheterization should apply sterile lubricant to the insertion end of the chosen catheter (with sterile, lubricated stylet already inserted, if used). If using a metal catheter, make certain the insertion end is tipped downward prior to insertion. Note if the metal catheter flange attachment corresponds to the side toward which the catheter insertion end is tipped or to the opposite side, since this will help the individual performing catheterization ensure that the insertion end remains tipped downward during the catheterization process. The insertion end of the lubricated catheter is advanced into the vulva and along the dorsal wall of the vestibule in an upward direction initially to attempt to bypass the clitoral fossa. After the initial dorsal advancement, the catheter should be directed more cranially, sliding the catheter gently toward the ventral surface of the vagina and observing

the external end of the catheter for the appearance of urine. If the catheter advances into the urethra and the bladder lumen, less resistance to advancement is often noted. If entry into the bladder lumen is suspected but no obvious urine flow is observed, a syringe should be attached to the flared end of the catheter (with stylet removed, if used) and aspiration performed to determine if urine can be obtained (Figure 1.38). Attaching a syringe to the external end of a metal catheter may require the use of flexible tubing as an adapter (see Figure 1.22). If no urine appears by natural flow or aspiration, the catheterization attempt can be continued either with the same catheter or a catheter of different composition and/or diameter. Access to the urethral orifice can sometimes be facilitated by lightly compressing the urinary bladder through the abdomen while advancing the catheter along the ventral vaginal wall. Over-insertion of the catheter should be avoided

5. If a stylet has been used in the catheterization process and is still in place, it should be removed once successful catheterization is believed to have been achieved

6. Ideally, a 5–10-mL sample of urine should be collected for submission by catching urine flowing freely out of the catheter into a suitable container or by aspirating the desired amount into a syringe attached to the external catheter end. If urine is flowing freely or can be aspirated after obtaining the initial sample, a second sample should be collected into a different container or syringe. If obtained, the second urine sample is the preferred sample for submission and analysis or culture since it has a lesser chance of contamination or collection artifact

7. Following completion of urine collection, the urinary catheter should be gently removed from the urogenital tract by steady withdrawal in a sterile manner

Feline Technique

1. Prepare for urine collection:
   a. Have one or two clean/sterile appropriate containers or syringes available for urine collection
   b. Select a suitable sterile urinary catheter appropriate in composition, size, and length for the patient (see text for guidelines). Sterile red rubber or other catheters of flexible materials and polypropylene catheters can be used in the transurethral catheterization of female cats. When more flexible catheters are used for the blind technique, it is often helpful to employ a lubricated stylet, giving added stiffness to the catheter in an attempt to facilitate tip insertion into the urethral orifice (Figure 1.39). Stainless steel catheters with angled insertion tips can also be advantageous in facilitating blind insertion, but must be used with the utmost care because of increased potential for urogenital trauma. Although the catheter selected should be of sufficient length to reach the bladder, the relatively short length of the urethra in the female cat generally permits transurethral catheterization using a standard "tomcat" catheter (approximately 3.5 Fr, 13 cm) (see Figure 1.19a). Longer catheters can be used but are not necessarily needed for short-term feline catheterization. If a longer catheter is used, care should be taken to prevent over-insertion so that complications, such as bladder trauma, urine collection impairment, and catheter retroflexion into the urethra, do not occur. Although the diameter of the feline urethra may accommodate a larger catheter than the 3.5 Fr size often chosen for short-term use, catheters larger in diameter can potentially produce more trauma to the urethra

    c. Sedation of the female feline patient is usually required for humane, successful transurethral catheterization

    d. Sterile gloves should be worn when performing this method of transurethral catheterization

2. Female cats are typically positioned in ventral recumbency. Using an assistant or mechanical restraint such as ties or an adhesive wrap, the tail should be positioned away from the area of the vulva. The hind limbs should be positioned in a flexed position alongside the body or, assuming the patient is sedated and has been placed on an elevated surface, can be allowed to hang downward from the supporting surface (see Figure 1.36a)

3. The vulva and adjacent skin should be cleaned with water, sterile sponges, and a disinfecting soap such as chlorhexidine, and then thoroughly rinsed to prevent both infection and iatrogenic changes in urinalysis results. Longer hair that may interfere with or contaminate the catheterization process may be clipped, if necessary

4. Wearing sterile gloves, the person performing catheterization should apply sterile lubricant to the insertion end of the chosen catheter (with sterile, lubricated stylet already inserted, if used). If using a metal catheter, make certain the insertion end is tipped downward prior to insertion. Note if the metal catheter flange attachment corresponds to the side toward which the catheter insertion end is tipped or to the opposite side, since this will help ensure that the insertion end remains tipped downward during the catheterization process. The insertion end of the lubricated catheter is advanced cranially through the vulva and vestibule into the vagina, observing the flared or external end of the catheter for the appearance of urine. If the catheter advances into the urethra and the bladder lumen, less resistance to advancement is often noted. If entry into the bladder lumen is suspected but no obvious urine flow is observed, a syringe should be attached to the flared or adapter end of the catheter (with stylet removed, if used) and aspiration performed to determine if urine can be obtained. If no urine appears by natural flow or aspiration, the catheterization attempt can be continued either with the same catheter or a catheter of different composition and/or diameter. Access to the urethral orifice can sometimes be facilitated by lightly compressing the bladder through the abdomen while advancing the catheter along the ventral vaginal wall. Over-insertion of the catheter should be avoided by discontinuing advancement of the catheter 1–2 cm after initial urine flow through the catheter has been observed

5. If a stylet has been used in the catheterization process and is still in place, it should be removed once successful catheterization has been achieved

6. Ideally, a 5–10-mL sample of urine should be collected for submission by catching urine flowing freely out of the catheter into a suitable container or by aspirating the desired amount into a syringe attached to the external catheter end. If urine is flowing freely or can be aspirated after obtaining the initial sample, a second sample should be collected into a different container or syringe. If obtained, the second urine sample is the preferred sample for submission and analysis or culture since it has a lesser chance of contamination or collection artifact

7. Following completion of urine collection, the urinary catheter should be gently removed from the urogenital tract by steady withdrawal in a sterile manner

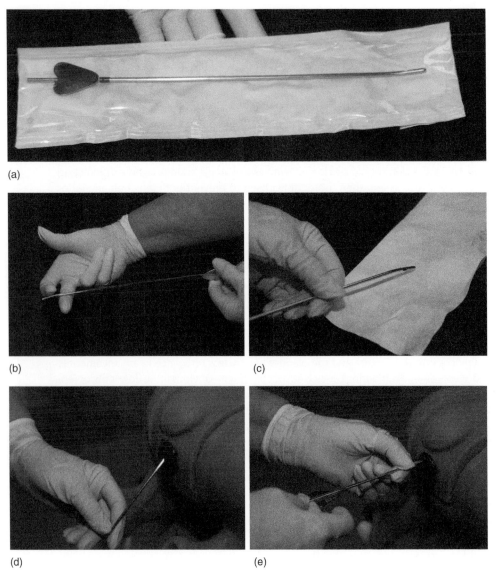

(a)

(b)   (c)

(d)   (e)

Figure 1.38 Demonstration of transurethral catheterization in a female dog by the blind method using a canine female catheterization mannequin positioned in ventral recumbency. (a) A stainless steel urinary catheter is chosen; note that the chosen catheter does not have a flared end for syringe attachment. (b) The position of flange attachment should also be noted; in the catheter pictured the side of flange attachment corresponds to the side toward which the insertion end of the catheter is tipped. (c) Sterile lubricant is applied to the insertion end of the selected catheter. (d) Wearing sterile gloves, the individual performing catheterization inserts the catheter (with the tip pointing downward) through the cleansed vulva and gently slides the catheter upward along the dorsal aspect of the vestibule. (e) When resistance is met after the initial dorsal advancement, the catheter should be directed gently cranially along the ventral aspect of the vagina, noting if less resistance is suddenly detected and if urine appears at the outer end of the catheter since these features indicate successful entry into the bladder lumen. It should also be noted in the metal catheter pictured that the flange attachment is on the down side of the catheter, indicating that the insertion end is tipped in the preferred downward position. If syringe attachment to the metal catheter is desired, flexible tubing can be attached to the outer catheter end, allowing a syringe to be connected for urine aspiration (see Figure 1.22).

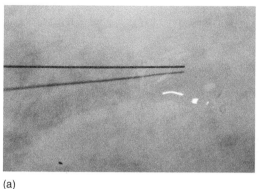

(a)

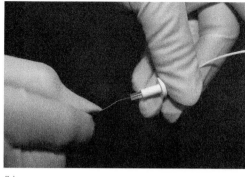

(b)

Figure 1.39 (a) Applying sterile lubricant to stylet to be inserted into selected catheter. (b) Inserting lubricated stylet into flexible tomcat catheter to provide added stiffness for blind transurethral catheterization.

Cystocentesis

Cystocentesis (Box 1.9) is a method of obtaining urine from the urinary bladder by means of transabdominal needle puncture. This urine collection technique is performed by trained personnel and is generally easy to carry out in small animals without sedation, especially with the assistance of ultrasonography. It is often the preferred technique when establishing the significance of cells or bacteria in a urine sample or when collecting urine for culture. When properly performed, there is a low risk of iatrogenic urinary tract infection. Surgical preparation of the abdominal skin site selected for needle penetration is not generally required, although removal of excessive hair and application of antiseptic solution is often recommended. Samples obtained via cystocentesis typically contain microscopic blood contamination, limiting the usefulness of this urine collection method for monitoring patients in which microscopic hematuria has been identified as the primary urinalysis abnormality. Additional drawbacks of cystocentesis include difficulty in sampling due to inadequate bladder urine volume, potential patient resistance to restraint and positioning, inadvertent intestinal or blood vessel sampling, urinary bladder laceration, induction of a vagal response, seeding of neoplastic cells along the needle path in patients with transitional cell carcinoma, and leakage of urine into the abdomen. The risk of bladder laceration and urine leakage is small unless the urinary bladder is over-distended or there is bladder wall pathology. This technique is generally contraindicated in animals with a coagulopathy or on anticoagulant therapy and should be used with caution in patients that have had recent cystotomy.

Using a 22- or 23-gauge needle 1–1.5 inches (2.5–3.8 cm) in length is generally preferred for obtaining a sample suitable for urinalysis or culture and minimizing the opportunity for undesirable consequences to the patient. In very large or obese patients a 3-inch (7.6-cm) 22-gauge spinal needle may be needed to reach the bladder (Figure 1.40). Although syringes used for cystocentesis to obtain diagnostic urine samples generally range from 3 to 12 mL, a 5-mL syringe is easily handled and usually of adequate volume to obtain a specimen suitable for most urinalysis evaluations.

Techniques for canine and feline cystocentesis using palpation, ultrasound-guided, and blind methods are described in Box 1.9 (Figures 1.41–1.44). The box includes technique modifications related to the species and sex of the patient.

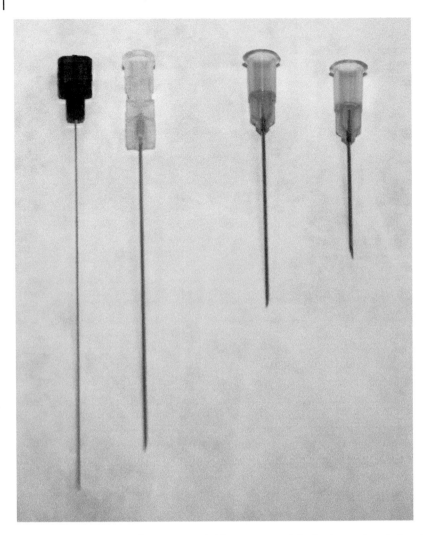

Figure 1.40 Needles typically recommended for cystocentesis in the dog and cat. Left to right: 22-gauge 2.5-inch spinal needle with stylet removed; 22-gauge 1.5-inch cystocentesis needle; 22-gauge 1-inch hypodermic needle.

Box 1.9 **Canine and feline cystocentesis techniques.**

---

1. Prepare for urine collection:
   a. Palpate the patient's abdomen to assess the degree of bladder distention and if any potentially complicating factors are present such as a palpable bladder mass suggestive of transitional cell carcinoma (increases patient risk for neoplastic cell seeding), nonpalpable or very small bladder volume (decreases chances for successful urine collection or may alter performance of cystocentesis technique), or a descending colon distended with feces (increases chance of inadvertent intestinal sampling, especially, in patients with small bladder volume). Ultrasonography may also be used to help determine the presence of complicating factors
   b. When the bladder is unable to be palpated and ultrasonography assistance is not an option, the patient can be hospitalized and cage confined until the bladder is distended sufficiently to be palpable. If hospitalization is not possible, the patient's physical characteristics make bladder palpation difficult, or pollakiuria makes it unlikely that the bladder will achieve palpable distention, the blind method of cystocentesis can be considered or a technique for urine collection other than cystocentesis can be chosen
   c. Have a suitable hypodermic/spinal needle, syringe, and a clean/sterile container appropriate for urine submission available. See the text for guidelines regarding appropriate needle and syringe selection. Box 9.1 point 4 provides some additional comments regarding the use of a spinal needle for cystocentesis. In some instances, especially when placing collected urine into culture tubes, it is beneficial to have an additional sterile hypodermic needle available for specimen transfer in order to decrease the possibility of specimen contamination by the needle used in obtaining the cystocentesis sample
   d. If ultrasonographic assistance in location and aspiration of the patient's bladder is anticipated, the ultrasound unit, transducer, and coupling gel (if used) should be readily available. A convex or curvilinear 5–7 MHz transducer is commonly used in performing cystocentesis
   e. Unless the patient is sedated/anesthetized, an assistant or assistants should be available to help in patient restraint for the procedure
2. Determine the cystocentesis technique to be used and position the patient appropriately for the procedure. The patient's temperament and size, ease of bladder palpation, presence of complicating factors, the necessity/availability of ultrasonographic assistance, and the availability of personnel for restraint are all factors which play a role in determining the method of cystocentesis and associated positioning of the patient. The patient can be placed in a standing, laterally recumbent, or dorsally recumbent position. All of these positions are common choices for patients undergoing cystocentesis by the bladder palpation method. Smaller patients or larger patients with distended bladders often have cystocentesis performed when in a standing or laterally recumbent position. A laterally or, frequently, dorsally recumbent position is the position of choice for patients undergoing ultrasound-assisted cystocentesis or patients requiring a greater degree of restraint for the cystocentesis procedure. Dorsal recumbency may be beneficial in obtaining a cystocentesis sample from patients with smaller, less palpable bladders and is the position of choice for performing cystocentesis by the blind technique. One assistant for restraint is generally adequate for a patient placed in a standing or laterally recumbent position (larger or agitated patients may require two assistants for adequate restraint). Patients placed in dorsal recumbency often require two assistants for restraint with one assistant restraining the head and front limbs and the second assistant extending the hind limbs away from the posterior abdomen (Figure 1.41)

3. Cystocentesis methods include:
   a. Bladder palpation method (see text for guidelines related to needle and syringe selection). After the patient has been positioned, the palpable bladder should be immobilized with one hand, pushing it gently dorsally and posteriorly. The anticipated area of needle insertion into the bladder is usually ventral or ventrolateral. The abdominal skin overlying the area of bladder puncture is often sparsely haired, but may be clipped, if necessary. The skin insertion site does not have to be surgically prepped, but should be moistened with alcohol or disinfectant, wetting down any hair in the area to enhance skin exposure. The hand which is not immobilizing the bladder should be used to insert the selected needle with attached syringe into the bladder through the abdominal wall. Ideally, when inserted through the abdomen, the needle should be posteriorly angled approximately 45° from the long axis of the patient. Angling the needle inserted not only helps maintain the needle in the bladder lumen but also reduces the possibility of urine leakage from the bladder into the abdomen (Figure 1.42)
   b. Ultrasound-guided method (see text and earlier in this box for guidelines related to needle, syringe, and ultrasound transducer selection). Ultrasound-guided cystocentesis is ideal to successfully obtain a urine sample with the least potential for undue patient trauma and blood or bowel contamination, especially in patients with minimal to moderate bladder distention. The patient is commonly placed in dorsal recumbency although lateral recumbency is also an option. If dorsally recumbent, the use of a foam trough can enhance patient comfort and positioning. The abdominal site for positioning of the transducer and needle is the posterior ventral or ventrolateral abdomen. Hair can be clipped, if needed. The selected site should be moistened with alcohol. Coupling gel can be applied directly to the transducer or conservatively to the selected skin site. Once the bladder has been located with the transducer an area directly adjacent to the tranducer should be cleaned of coupling gel, if used, and moistened with alcohol. The needle selected for cystocentesis with syringe attached should be inserted through the cleaned skin site and directed to the bladder, taking care to keep the needle tip within the plane of the ultrasound beam so that insertion into the bladder can be observed (Figure 1.43)
   c. Blind method (see text for guidelines related to needle and syringe selection). In the blind cystocentesis technique the canine or feline patient is positioned in dorsal recumbency, and an area on the abdominal midline halfway between the umbilicus and the pelvic brim is selected for insertion of the selected needle (typically 22-gauge, 1–1.5-inch) with an attached syringe. Alternatively, in the female dog and the male or female cat, the needle insertion site can be determined by dripping alcohol on the posterior ventral midline and observing the midline point at which the alcohol pools. The point of alcohol pooling is more easily assessed in patients with lesser amounts of hair obscuring the midline and trapping the dripped alcohol. Blind cystocentesis approximates a point in the abdomen where, at least, a portion of the bladder is frequently located. Prior to needle insertion the site should be moistened with alcohol or, if alcohol was pooled to select the site, excess alcohol should be absorbed with a clean cotton ball. Unlike the other variations of cystocentesis technique described in this box, needle insertion in blind cystocentesis is usually perpendicular to the long axis of the patient rather than at a more acute angle (Figure 1.44). When inserting the needle and attached syringe in the male dog, the prepuce and penis are pushed laterally to allow unhindered access to the patient's midline. Without the input of palpation or ultrasound, the depth of needle insertion is dependent upon the length of the needle and the body condition of the patient. It should be remembered that the blind cystocentesis method has the highest risk of the three cystocentesis methods described here for causing complications, such as sample contamination and injury to the patient

4. When a spinal needle is chosen for the cystocentesis procedure, the stylet which usually accompanies the needle can often be removed and the needle inserted with syringe attached in the manner previously described for the various cystocentesis methods. However, if more resistance to insertion is anticipated due to the condition of the skin at the site of insertion, the stylet can be left in place until abdominal penetration has occurred, to provide more needle stability and decrease the chances of obstructing the needle with tissue or blood. Following penetration, the stylet can be removed and the syringe for aspiration quickly attached to the needle hub to limit the introduction of any free air into the abdominal cavity. Insertion of the spinal needle into the urinary bladder lumen can then proceed

5. Regardless of any technique variations, once needle penetration into the bladder lumen is believed to have occurred, negative pressure should be applied to the syringe attached to the insertion needle. Aspiration should continue until the desired amount of urine is obtained (5 mL is considered the ideal minimum amount for standard urinalysis), urine flow stops, or frank blood or no urine appears in the syringe barrel. Recommendations for these outcomes are as follows:

   a. Adequate urine sample obtained: stop applying negative pressure and withdraw needle from the abdomen

   b. Inadequate or no urine sample obtained: negative pressure is discontinued. The needle can be moved slightly outward or inward in a direct line with the insertion angle and then aspiration can again be attempted. Frequently, if re-aspiration is attempted, the needle is totally withdrawn from the abdomen and then re-inserted in a position and angle suggested by the palpation or ultrasound information available. When performing cystocentesis by the blind method, re-insertion of the needle through the abdomen should occur slightly cranial or caudal to the original midline insertion point. *The insertion needle should never be re-directed from one angle to another while located in the bladder regardless of how cystocentesis is attempted. Re-direction when the needle is in the abdomen but outside the bladder can be cautiously attempted with the assistance of ultrasonography.* Three unsuccessful attempts to obtain an adequate urine sample using any of the cystocentesis methods should cause further cystocentesis attempts to be delayed until the bladder becomes more distended with urine and consideration should be given to alternative means of obtaining a urine sample

   c. Frank blood appears: discontinue aspiration attempts. Observe the patient for any signs of weakness, pale mucous membranes, or other signs of patient instability. Abdominal ultrasonography can also be considered to check for accumulation of abdominal fluid. Wait at least 24–48 hours prior to re-attempting cystocentesis or attempting urine collection by a different technique

6. Negative pressure should always be discontinued when withdrawing the insertion needle from the bladder and abdomen. Excessive pressure on the bladder should be avoided when using palpation as part of the cystocentesis technique or in the immediate post-cystocentesis period regardless of the method used, in order to minimize the possibility of urine leakage from the bladder

7. The urine obtained by cystocentesis should be submitted in a timely manner and in an appropriate container for the desired analyses

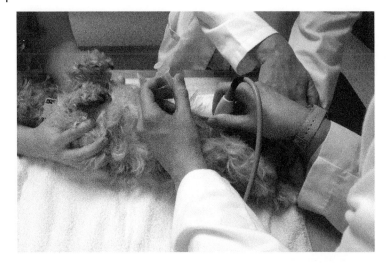

Figure 1.41 Restraint for cystocentesis when the patient is dorsally recumbent usually requires two assistants, one for restraint of the head and front limbs and one for caudal extension of the hind limbs away from the abdomen.

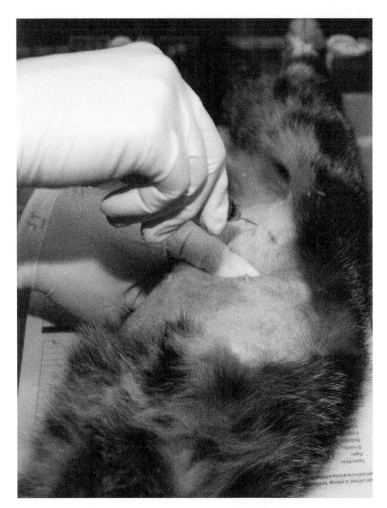

Figure 1.42 Cystocentesis by bladder palpation method. The cat is placed in dorsal recumbency. The bladder is immobilized by pushing the bladder posteriorly and dorsally with one hand while the other hand directs a 22-gauge needle with syringe attached through the alcohol-moistened ventral abdominal wall at a 45° angle to the long axis of the patient. Although the patient's abdomen has been shaved and the individual performing the cystocentesis is wearing gloves, neither of these components is required to perform the procedure.

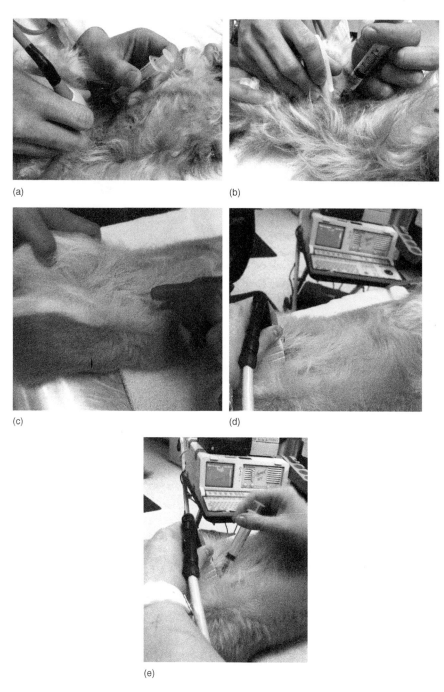

Figure 1.43 Cystocentesis performed by the ultrasound-guided method. (a) An ultrasound transducer is used to locate the urinary bladder in a dorsally recumbent canine patient with sparse abdominal hair. (b) The selected needle with syringe attached punctures the abdominal wall adjacent to the transducer and is guided to the bladder for urine aspiration, taking care to keep the needle tip within the ultrasound beam. (c) Alcohol is sprayed on the abdomen of a dorsally recumbent canine patient with a denser hair coat than the patient pictured in (a) and (b). (d) The ultrasound screen can be seen as the transducer is used to locate the urinary bladder in the area of the posterior abdomen. (e) When the urinary bladder has been located with the transducer, the selected needle with syringe attached punctures the abdominal wall adjacent to the transducer and is guided to the bladder for urine aspiration, keeping the needle tip within the ultrasound beam.

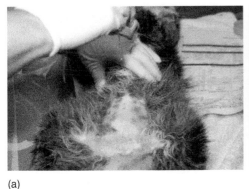
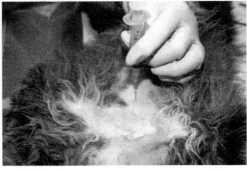

(a)   (b)

Figure 1.44 (a) Alcohol is dripped on the shaved abdominal midline of a cat in dorsal recumbency to observe the point of alcohol pooling and locate a transabdominal needle insertion site for blind cystocentesis. (b) A 22-gauge hypodermic needle with a 6-mL syringe attached is inserted through the midline abdominal wall and perpendicular to the long axis of the cat's body at the site of alcohol pooling as part of the blind cystocentesis technique.

Urine Sample Handling

Urine samples should be examined within 1 hour after collection to avoid artifactual changes. If the urine cannot be examined within that time period or is to be shipped to a commercial laboratory, it can be refrigerated with a tightly secured lid (Figure 1.45) for up to 6 hours. If the sample is sent to a commercial laboratory, sending the urine sample with a cold pack may delay the onset of some artifactual changes (Box 1.10). Urine samples submitted to a diagnostic laboratory for cytologic evaluation should be sent in an EDTA tube (see Figure 1.3) to delay cell deterioration and prevent the overgrowth of bacteria (if urine culture is desired some urine should be submitted in a clean, sterile container with no additives or in culture tubes as EDTA can inhibit the growth of some bacteria and the tubes may not be sterile). Cells in urine deteriorate rapidly and the evaluation of cellular morphology is best accomplished using fresh urine samples; therefore, it is always prudent to include one or two air-dried urine sediment slides.

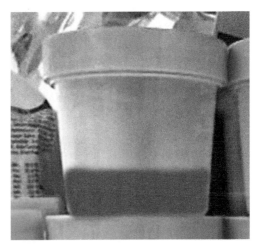

Figure 1.45 If a urine sample cannot be analyzed within 1 hour after collection, the sample should be refrigerated in a suitable container with a tightly secured lid.

Culture

Cystocentesis is the preferred collection method when evaluating urine for evidence of infection, including submission of a sample for culture. When a urine sample obtained by cystocentesis is transferred to a container appropriate for culture, the needle which was used to obtain the sample should be discarded and a new, sterile hypodermic needle should be used for transfer to the culture tube. Although catheterized or free-catch, midstream, voided or manually expressed samples can be used in determining the presence of urinary tract infection (UTI),

Box 1.10 **Changes in urine samples from delayed processing.**

Color change
Increased odor
Increased turbidity
Increased pH
Decreased glucose
Decreased ketones
Decreased bilirubin
Decreased cellularity
Increase or decrease in number of crystals (dependent on type, temperature, and urine pH)
Deterioration of casts
Deterioration of cells
Deterioration of crystals
Increased bacterial growth at room temperature
Decreased bacterial growth with prolonged refrigeration

urine collected by these methods is subject to contamination from the genital tract, skin, and hair. The potential for bacterial contamination is particularly high in urine samples collected by voiding or manual compression even when a midstream specimen has been collected. Consequently, submission of midstream voided or manually compressed urine samples for culture is not routinely recommended.

Regardless of the urine collection technique, diagnosis of UTI through urinalysis and culture is best determined when the patient undergoing evaluation has not received antimicrobial therapy for at least 3–5 days prior to sample collection. Cultures should be performed immediately after urine collection, although this is seldom practical unless in-house agar plating of the collected urine sample is possible. In most circumstances urine will be sent to a diagnostic laboratory. Urine should be placed in a sterile container, with a tightly secured lid, and placed in the refrigerator within 30 minutes of collection; ideally, culture should be performed on the refrigerated sample within 12 hours of collection. Some organisms may be killed with prolonged refrigeration. Freezing urine samples may kill bacteria. When submitting a urine sample for culture to a laboratory, consider saving and sending the sample in

a preservative tube (see Figure 1.4a), which can aid in stabilizing organism content of the urine specimen for up to 72 hours post-collection without refrigeration (see Box 1.1). Preservative tubes help maintain original pathogen numbers, decrease proliferation of contaminant organisms, and allow time for evaluation of concurrent diagnostic procedures prior to culture submission. Urine submitted in EDTA is not appropriate for culture as EDTA can inhibit the growth of some bacteria and the tubes may not be sterile.

To be an effective diagnostic and therapeutic tool, urine culture should be evaluated in conjunction with the following information:

- patient signalment, history, and physical findings;
- method of urine collection;
- specific identification of the cultured organism(s);
- quantitative bacterial numbers of the cultured organism(s);
- antimicrobial susceptibility testing of the cultured organism(s);
- results of urinalysis and other indicated diagnostic procedures.

Knowledge of patient signalment, history, and physical findings can raise the index of suspicion that UTI exists, identify predisposing causes, help localize the site of potential infection, and determine further diagnostic procedures. Knowledge of urine collection method is important due to the potential for microorganism contamination. Identification and/or quantification of organisms help establish the presence of UTI, give an indication of whether the organisms represent reinfection versus relapse in patients with a history of multiple UTI episodes, and help direct therapy.

Bacterial quantification in conjunction with knowledge of the urine collection technique can assist in verifying UTI versus contamination, given that bacterial numbers in colony-forming units per milliliter (CFU/mL) have been established for the various collection methods and likelihood of canine and feline UTI (Lulich and Osborne, 1999). In general, lower bacterial numbers from urine culture are most likely to be representative of true UTI when the sample has been collected by cystocentesis ($\geq$1000 CFU/mL, cat and dog) rather than by catheterization ($\geq$10 000 CFU/mL, dog and $\geq$1000 CFU/mL, cat) or midstream voided and manual compression techniques ($\geq$100 000 CFU/mL, dog and $\geq$10 000 CFU/mL, cat). Bacterial numbers from urine culture most compatible with contamination have been reported as $\leq$100 CFU/mL (dog and cat) for cystocentesis samples, $\leq$1000 CFU/mL (dog) and $\leq$100 CFU/mL (cat) for catheterized samples, and $\leq$10 000 CFU/mL (dog) and $\leq$1000 CFU/mL (cat) for midstream voided and manual expression samples. It should be noted that cats are more resistant to UTI than dogs and lower bacterial numbers from urine culture may have more significance in terms of indication of infection for cats in contrast to dogs. In any case, the significance of quantified bacterial culture results should always be interpreted in conjunction with the other evaluation aspects listed above. Antimicrobial susceptibility testing is essential for establishing an appropriate therapeutic regimen. Although UTI can be present without the identification of inflammatory cells on urinalysis, the presence of inflammatory cells increases the probability that bacteria observed on urinalysis and/or culture are truly associated with UTI. Additional diagnostic procedures performed on patients with suspected UTI, such as diagnostic imaging and biochemistry profiles, can help provide further evidence of UTI, identify complicating factors, and help localize the site of infection.

2

Initial Assessment: Physical Characteristics

Volume

In health, urine output is influenced by several elements (nutritional and water content in food and free water intake). The normal urine output for dogs and cats is 20–45 mL/kg/day.

Color

Urine is normally a pale yellow, yellow, or an amber color (Figure 2.1). The shade and intensity of the color are most commonly determined by a combination of urine volume and concentration as well as the amount of the endogenous pigments, urochrome and urobilin. Abnormal urine color may occur for a variety of reasons, such as health, diet, medications, and environment. These influences can result in variations of the usual color determinants, including the type and amount of both endogenous and exogenous pigments found in the urine. Excessive or abnormal urine pigment may interfere with the ability of the examiner to interpret urine chemistry reagent strip results accurately. Gradations of red to brown (Figures 2.2, 2.3) are the most common abnormal colors observed in patients and can be associated with multiple causes but are usually related to hematuria (red blood cells [RBCs] in the urine), hemoglobinuria, bilirubinuria, or myoglobinuria. Consequently, urine samples with a red or brown hue should prompt reagent dipstick testing for bilirubin and occult

blood, and urine sediment examination for RBCs (Figure 2.4). Occasionally, other urine colors can be associated with bilirubinuria, hemoglobinuria, myoglobinuria, and/or hematuria, including green, orange, or black.

Variations in color can also be the result of urine sediment components other than RBCs, such as lipids, white blood cells (WBCs), and crystals, which can occasionally produce a white, milky urine. It is possible for urine to take on an unusually dark yellow to brownish-yellow color as a normal manifestation of the typical endogenous pigments, urochrome and urobilin, when the patient has very concentrated urine. Although infrequent, atypical components can sometimes result in discoloration of urine which may be mistaken for hematuria or other familiar medical conditions. Pseudohematuria is the term applied to urine discoloration, most commonly red to brown hues, produced by such atypical components. These unusual components are generally endogenous or exogenous pigments (Bartges, 2005) which can be derived from genetic conditions such as porphyria, drugs (e.g. doxorubicin), food dyes, and toxins (e.g. mercury). When routine urine chemistry and sediment findings cannot provide a satisfactory explanation for urine discoloration, the history and physical findings of the patient should be reviewed and further diagnostic procedures considered (see Figure 2.4). State veterinary diagnostic laboratories and university-associated medical genetic facilities (e.g. PennGen) can

Atlas of Canine and Feline Urinalysis, First Edition. Theresa E. Rizzi, Amy Valenciano, Mary Bowles, Rick Cowell, Ronald Tyler, and Dennis B. DeNicola.
© 2017 John Wiley & Sons, Inc. Published 2017 by John Wiley & Sons, Inc.

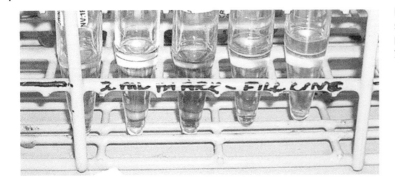

Figure 2.1 All the urine samples are clear. Colors are pale yellow, amber, and yellow.

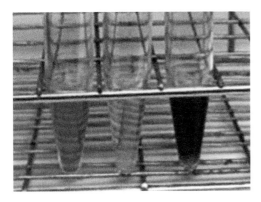

Figure 2.2 Amber, yellow, and brown urine (left to right).

serve as valuable resources for information and diagnostic testing related to cases of suspected pseudohematuria.

Clarity/Turbidity

The physical property of turbidity refers to the degree of clarity of the urine and is generally reported in a range from clear to flocculent. Normal urine is usually described as clear to very mildly cloudy (Figure 2.5; see Figure 2.1). Turbidity most often correlates to the amount of particulate matter present in the urine in the form of cells, crystals, amorphous debris, lipid, microorganisms, and mucus. Occasionally, semen and feces can also contribute to turbidity. The cause of turbidity is usually determined by microscopic examination of urine sediment.

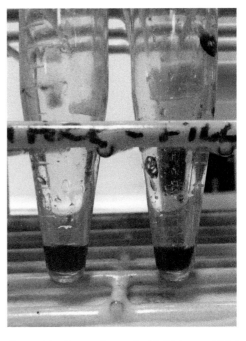

Figure 2.3 Urine sediment. Red (left), brown (right) urine should prompt dipstick colorimetric testing for bilirubin and occult blood.

Odor

Urine typically does not have a strong odor, but odor is affected by urine concentration, diet, medications, the presence of bacteria, inflammation, and certain medical conditions (e.g. in diabetes mellitus, a sweet or fruity urine odor is sometimes detected). Improperly stored or aged samples may have a stronger odor.

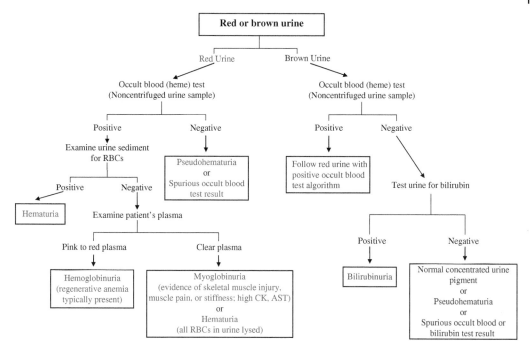

Red or brown urine

Red Urine — Brown Urine

Occult blood (heme) test
(Noncentrifuged urine sample)

Occult blood (heme) test
(Noncentrifuged urine sample)

Positive — Negative

Positive — Negative

Examine urine sediment
for RBCs

Pseudohematuria
or
Spurious occult blood
test result

Follow red urine with
positive occult blood
test algorithm

Test urine for bilirubin

Positive — Negative

Hematuria

Examine patient's plasma

Pink to red plasma — Clear plasma

Positive — Negative

Hemoglobinuria
(regenerative anemia
typically present)

Myoglobinuria
(evidence of skeletal muscle injury,
muscle pain, or stiffness; high CK, AST)
or
Hematuria
(all RBCs in urine lysed)

Bilirubinuria

Normal concentrated urine
pigment
or
Pseudohematuria
or
Spurious occult blood or
bilirubin test result

Figure 2.4 Diagnostic algorithm for red or brown urine. AST, aspartate aminotransferase; CK, creatine kinase. *Source:* Adapted from Bowles MH, Lorenz MD. *Small Animal Medical Diagnosis* 3rd edn. Wiley-Blackwell, 2009; pp. 258–273.

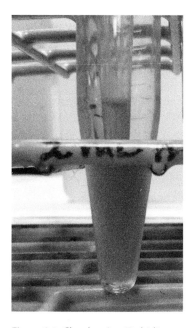

Figure 2.5 Cloudy urine. Turbidity correlates to the amount of particulate matter present in the urine

Urine Specific Gravity

Urine specific gravity (USG), measured with a refractometer (Figure 2.6), is an indirect measurement of urine osmolality. The interpretation of USG is dependent on several factors, such as hydration status, electrolyte concentrations, serum creatinine and urea nitrogen

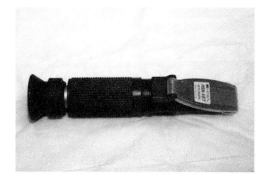

Figure 2.6 Hand-held veterinary refractometer used for measuring urine specific gravity.

Table 2.1 Causes of polydypsia/polyuria in the dog and cat.

Endocrine disorders	Electrolyte/mineral imbalance	Urologic disorders	Iatrogenic/drug-related	Miscellaneous
Acromegaly	Hypercalcemia	Chronic or acute renal disease*	Alcohol	Diet
Central diabetes insipidus	Hyperkalemia	Fanconi syndrome	Drugs	Excessive vitamin D
Diabetes mellitus	Hypokalemia	Postobstructive diuresis	Antiepileptics	Increased NaCl
Hyperadrenocorticism	Hyponatremia	Congenital nephrogenic diabetes insipidus	Dextrose	Ultra-low protein
Hyperthyroidism			Diuretics	Hepatic failure
Hypoadrenocorticism			Glucocorticoids	Paraneoplastic syndrome (e.g. tumor may induce hypercalcemia and/or 2° NDI**)
Pheochromocytoma		Primary renal glycosuria	Vitamin D	Polycythemia
Primary hyperaldosteronism		Pyelonephritis	Fluid therapy	Portosystemic shunt
Primary hyperparathyroidism		Renal medullary washout	NaCl	Psychogenic (primary) polydipsia
				2° NDI**
				Splenomegaly (Nelson and Couto, 2003)

*PD/PU most common in chronic renal disease.

**2° NDI = secondary (acquired) nephrogenic diabetes insipidus, a condition which can be induced by the majority of causes of PD/PU listed.

concentrations, the administration of certain medications (corticosteroids, diuretics, antiepileptics), and the administration of fluid therapy. In addition, there are some clinical entities which hinder the kidneys' ability to concentrate urine, particularly conditions that cause polydipsia (water intake greater than $100\,mL/kg/day$) and polyuria (urine output greater than $50\,mL/kg/day$). Causes of polydipsia/polyuria in the dog and cat typically result in patient USGs less than 1.025 (Table 2.1). It should also be recognized that any factors which contribute to elevations of NaCl, glucose, or protein in the urine can result in a related increase in USG. As a consequence of the multiple factors influencing USG and its interpretation, the "normal" reference intervals often listed for USG (Dog: 1.015–1.045; Cat: 1.035–1.060) can be misleading.

Hyposthenuria refers to USG less than 1.007. This is dilute urine indicating specific gravity lower than that of plasma and glomerular filtrate. *Isosthenuria* refers to a USG between 1.008 and 1.013, equal to that of plasma and glomerular filtrate. A dehydrated animal with normal renal function will be able to avidly resorb water which will result in increased USG and reduced urine output. Demonstration of adequate urine concentrating ability is typically associated with a USG ≥ 1.040 in the cat and >1.030 in the dog. The USG representing maximum urine concentration in cats is 1.085 and 1.070 in dogs (Osborne and Stevens, 1999).

Refractometers are calibrated for the urine constituents of different species and therefore each calibration scale will be negligibly different in most species. Medical refractometers used for humans falsely increase urine specific gravity in feline patients. While the difference is negligible at USG <1.015, the discrepancy increases when USG >1.025 (George, 2001). There are many types of refractometers available, including digital. Using a hand-held refractometer, a single drop of urine is placed on the glass surface under the plastic cover. While the examiner is looking through the eye piece, the refractometer is held up to a light source and the USG is recorded at the light/dark interface on the scale. Digital refractometers will automatically display the urine specific gravity once the urine sample has been introduced into the instrument according to manufacturer instructions.

3

Urine Chemistry

The urine chemistry analysis is performed using commercially available urine chemistry test strips impregnated with colorimetric reagents (dipstick colorimetric test or DSCT) (Figure 3.1). Change in reagent color corresponds with the presence of the substance that the test strip is designed to detect. The intensity of the color change is proportional to the concentration of the substance being measured. Color changes may be subtle and individual visual acuity for color determination can vary, leading to variations in assessment among individuals. Several semi-automated instruments are commercially available for reading reagent test strips. This technology is based on the principle of reflectance; the amount of light reflected is inversely proportional to the concentration of the substance present.

There are several multiple-reagent test strips commercially available for use in humans and animals. These test strips differ only in the number of tests available on the strip and in the reagents used in the reagent pads. Since some of the test pads are not useful or reliable in animal species, some manufacturers of veterinary urine chemistry test strips exclude those tests. The use of test strips primarily manufactured for human urine testing is acceptable; however the test pads for urine specific gravity, urobilinogen, nitrite, and leukocyte esterase are not reliable for veterinary patients. The use of the urine chemistry multi-test strips is simple and, when the manufacturer's recommendations are followed, these tests usually provide reliable screening information. Following the manufacturer's recommendations includes adhering to the dipping method described in the instructions accompanying the test strips. Dropping urine on the test strip pads will not provide accurate results in some test strips which require full immersion of the strip into the urine sample being analyzed (Figure 3.2).

Urine pH

The test pad estimates pH (the concentration of hydrogen ions) of the urine using methyl red and bromthymol blue indicator dyes. The color changes correlate to the pH, ranging from 5.0 (acidic) to 9.0 (alkaline) in 0.5 pH unit increments. The pH value obtained by the DSCT is semiquantitative and is subject to the individual examiner's interpretation when not read by an automated instrument. One study comparing methods of urine pH measurement in dogs indicated that dipstick measurement of pH resulted in overestimation of the pH value (Johnson et al., 2007). Although not always critical, this overestimation tendency when using the DSCT could be more of an issue when a urine sample with a relatively neutral pH is falsely read as mildly alkaline, especially when monitoring pH for therapeutic purposes. Consequently, using a pH meter should be considered for patients where urine pH is felt to be a more critical value. The use of a pH meter need

Atlas of Canine and Feline Urinalysis, First Edition. Theresa E. Rizzi, Amy Valenciano, Mary Bowles, Rick Cowell, Ronald Tyler, and Dennis B. DeNicola.
© 2017 John Wiley & Sons, Inc. Published 2017 by John Wiley & Sons, Inc.

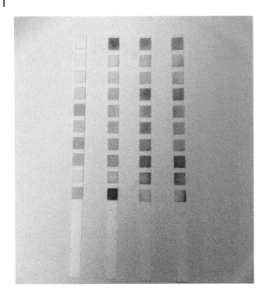

Figure 3.1 Dipstick colorimetric test strips used to perform urine chemistry analysis.

not be restricted to a commercial laboratory setting, since affordable handheld pH meters are available to the practitioner.

It is important to remember that urine pH can alter the results of urine sediment examination. Alkaline urine can cause crystal formation, notably precipitation of struvite crystals. Alkaline urine, especially specimens with a pH >8, can result in the disintegration of RBCs and WBCs as well as casts.

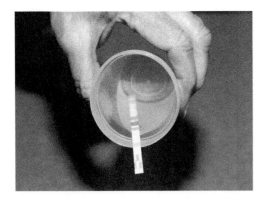

Figure 3.2 Full immersion into the urine sample is required for accurate results with some commercial multi-reagent urine test strips.

Cats and dogs typically have a urine pH in the range of 6.0–7.5; however, urine pH is affected by several factors, including delays in performing the chemistry analysis of urine samples. Following collection, carbon dioxide will diffuse out of the sample over time, increasing the pH of the urine specimen. In health, urine pH is chiefly influenced by diet. Animals that consume animal-protein-based diets (cats, dogs) have more acidic urine compared with animals that consume a plant- or vegetable-based diet (horses, ruminants), whose urine pH is more alkaline (7.5–8.5). Renal tubular disorders can interfere with the patient's ability to regulate hydrogen and bicarbonate ions, altering urine pH values. With systemic illness, the urine pH may indirectly reflect the overall acid–base status of the patient, as the kidneys compensate for systemic pH changes by varying the amount of hydrogen ions excreted. Consequently, patients with metabolic acidosis tend to acidify the urine, while patients with metabolic alkalosis tend to alkalinize the urine. However, overall acid–base status of the patient is still best determined by blood gas analysis. Alterations in urine pH can also occur in animals with urinary tract infections caused by bacteria that produce urease, resulting in the conversion of urea to ammonia with a subsequent increase in urine pH.

Protein

The urine protein pad contains pH-based indicator dye at acidic pH and, when bound to the amino groups of negatively charged proteins, it changes color. This is known as the "protein error of indicators" and is based on the ability of protein to alter the color of some acid–base indicators without altering the pH of the urine. The degree of color change corresponds to the estimated concentration of protein present. This method is more sensitive to albumin than to globulins, hemoglobin, myoglobin, Bence-Jones proteins (immunoglobin light chains), and mucoproteins, detecting as little as 5 mg albumin/dL urine on some test strips. A negative reaction is usually reliable which makes the DSCT for protein a good screening test. Because the DSCT protein pad is buffered to run the reaction at a very acidic pH, alkaline urine, especially urine with a pH of 8 or above, can overwhelm the buffer system in the protein pad and cause the reaction to run at a more alkaline pH, causing false increases in urine protein results.

There is usually little to no protein present in the urine. While glomerular filtration does not normally allow the passage of albumin and globulins, some smaller plasma proteins are freely filtered. These smaller proteins are routinely reabsorbed in the proximal tubules of the kidneys unless the concentration of these proteins overwhelms reabsorption or there is impairment of the renal tubules. Causes of proteinuria are listed in Table 3.1. Persistent proteinuria, especially without an obvious nonglomerular cause, should be diagnostically pursued.

Results of the urine test pad are often interpreted in conjunction with the urine specific gravity because the concentration of the urine protein is closely associated with the concentration or dilution of the urine. For example, a 2+ protein test pad result with a urine specific gravity of 1.010 constitutes a greater renal loss of protein than a 2+ protein result with a urine specific gravity of 1.030.

A positive reaction on the test pad ranges from trace, corresponding to 5–20 mg/dL depending on the test pad used, to 4+ which corresponds to greater than 1000 mg/dL of protein. False-positive test results often occur in mature feline patients due to the presence of cauxin (a peptidase) in feline urine. The protein test pad may be associated with the most errors in interpretation, as color changes on the test pad are subtle. In addition, any abnormal urine color may obscure the test pad color result. A variety of factors may cause the protein test pad to register either a false-positive or a false-negative result. These factors are listed in Table 3.2. When a false-positive result is suspected, the urine sample in question should be rechecked after eliminating the confounding factor, if possible, or another method of protein determination should be employed, such as the sulfosalicylic acid (SSA) turbidity test, chemical protein concentration determination, or a urine protein/creatinine ratio (UP:UC).

The SSA test is semiquantitative and performed by adding equal amounts of urine to a 5% solution of sulfosalicylic acid. The

Table 3.1 Causes of proteinuria.

Nonglomerular causes of proteinuria	
Urinary tract infection or inflammation	Common cause of proteinuria due to addition of inflammatory proteins and erythrocytes from the urinary or genital tract
Hemorrhage	Can originate anywhere along the urogenital tract. Erythrocytes and leukocytes present in the urinary sediment examination
Renal tubule damage (chronic renal disease, acute renal tubule damage)	Tubular proteinuria: small proteins that normally pass into the glomerular filtrate are either not reabsorbed or inadequately reabsorbed by damaged renal tubules
Hemoglobin, myoglobin, Bence-Jones proteins	Prerenal, overload or preglomerular proteinuria: high concentrations of these proteins in the blood result in high concentrations in the glomerular filtrate, overwhelming renal tubule resorptive capabilities
Glomerular causes of proteinuria	
Glomerular disease (glomerulonephritis, amyloidosis)	Often severe protein loss from the body, most significantly albumin, and other larger proteins
Physiologic	Functional proteinuria: transient increase in glomerular permeability to plasma proteins due to stress, temperature extremes (environmental or pyrexia), strenuous exercise, seizures, or venous congestion

Table 3.2 Factors capable of producing false dipstick urine protein results.

False-positive results	False-negative results
Alkaline urine pH (usually ≥ 8)	Very dilute urine
	Very acidic urine
Urine contaminants such as disinfectants or drug metabolites	Extremely small amounts of urine protein
Excessive urine contact time with protein test pad	Urine protein with low numbers of free amino groups (e.g. Bence-Jones proteins)

presence of proteins results in increased turbidity of the solution, which is evaluated on a trace to 4+ scale. Although the SSA test is most sensitive to albumin (sensitivity level >5 mg/dL), this test can detect the presence of globulins and Bence-Jones proteins. The SSA test should always be performed on the supernatant of centrifuged samples to avoid any initial sample turbidity that could make the interpretation of results difficult. False-positives can occur in patients with urine containing contrast media and high levels of β-lactam antibiotics, and false-negatives can sometimes occur with dilute urine samples. The SSA test was routinely performed by many laboratories to confirm the presence of protein indicated by DSCT screening, especially, in samples with an alkaline pH. However, based on more recently published (Welles et al., 2006) and unpublished (Fry, 2011) data, which indicated that the DSCT has equal specificity and equal or higher sensitivity for canine and feline proteinuria when compared to SSA results, quantitative urine protein concentration used in determining the urine protein to creatinine ratio (UP:UC) is currently recommended over the SSA test for confirmation and further assessment of proteinuria.

Quantitative measurement of urine protein concentration is accomplished via chemistry analyzer. The ratio derived by division of the urine protein concentration in mg/dL by the urine creatinine concentration in mg/dL

is the means by which the UP:UC is determined and is the most practical, accurate method for critical assessment of patient proteinuria. The quantitative measurement used in UP:UC determination can detect both albumin and globulins. The UP:UC has a greater sensitivity for urine protein detection (<5 mg/dL) than the DSCT. Most screening methods for the detection of proteinuria are affected by the urine volume and specific gravity. The UP:UC is unaffected by urine volume or specific gravity and, unlike the older 24-hour urine collection analyzer protein measurement, offers the additional benefit of providing accurate assessment from a single, random, midstream free-catch or cystocentesis sample. The reliability of the UP:UC is associated with the fact that protein and creatinine are handled similarly in patients with a stable glomerular filtration rate (GFR). Consequently, a patient with an unstable GFR, which is often the case in acute renal failure, is not a good candidate for proteinuria assessment via the UP:UC. Reliability of the UP:UC is also adversely affected by the presence of an active urine sediment (inflammation) or hyperproteinemia greater than 9 g/dL, both of which can make interpretation of UP:UC values difficult by contributing to the urine protein content of the sample. Although RBCs in the urine and the serum protein accompanying them can also cause an increase in the UP:UC values, only urine samples grossly affected by hemorrhage (i.e. red-tinged or overtly bloody) are likely to create notable elevations in UP:UC results. Mild increases in the UP:UC have sometimes been noted in patients receiving immunosuppressive doses of corticosteroids over a period of several weeks. A decrease in the UP:UC value can be seen in patients experiencing azotemia, since increasing blood creatinine concentration will result in increased tubular secretion of creatinine which, in turn, will increase urine creatinine and cause the UP:UC to be lowered. Although the UP:UC can be used to detect proteinuria, its value lies more in recognizing glomerular disease, as a monitor of therapeutic response, and as a prognostic indicator. Within the guidelines previously stated for reliable use of the UP:UC, an elevated ratio is a strong indicator of glomerular disease. Decreasing UP:UC values generally indicate positive response to therapy for conditions associated with proteinuria as long as the patient is not becoming progressively more azotemic. Finally, in a dog or cat with chronic renal disease, elevated or increasing UP:UC values are an indication that the patient is at greater risk for morbidity and mortality. Tables 3.3 and 3.4 provide numerical guidelines for UP:UC interpretation and related recommendations.

The microalbuminuria (MA) test is a more recent addition to the methods available for protein detection, specifically albumin. An in-house test is available (Heska's ERD-Screen^{TM} Urine Test) which diminishes the problem of measuring urine protein concentration in specimens of varying specific gravity by a standardization process prior to measurement of protein. The MA test is species-specific for the dog and cat and is more sensitive than either the DSCT or the SSA turbidometric test, detecting albumin concentrations from 1–30 mg/dL. The basic

Table 3.3 UP:UC interpretation and associated recommendations for canine patients with suspected or confirmed proteinuria.

Value	Interpretation	Recommendation
Nonazotemic dogs		
<0.5	WNRI	Monitor patient with suspected proteinuria by performing DSCT, SSA, MA, and/or UP:UC every 2–4 weeks for at least two times to document if proteinuria exists/persists Other diagnostic tests as indicated
0.5–1.0	Suspicious for renal proteinuria	Monitor patient by performing UP:UC periodically to confirm persistent renal proteinuria (three elevated UP:UC values found at ≥2-week intervals and not attributable to a prerenal or postrenal cause) or to identify progression of proteinuria Review history and physical findings; other diagnostic tests as indicated
>1.0	Abnormal	Review history and physical findings Perform diagnostic tests such as database, urogenital imaging, and urine culture Treat any underlying causes identified and monitor patient
≥2.0	High probability of glomerular proteinuria (may be tubular proteinuria [range 1–5])	Review history and physical findings Perform diagnostic tests such as database, urogenital imaging, and urine culture Treat any underlying causes identified Initiate renoprotective therapeutic intervention$^\alpha$ if persistent renal proteinuria identified Monitor patient appropriately
>5	Most commonly associated with glomerular disorders (glomerulonephritis or amyloidosis)	Review history and physical findings Perform diagnostic tests such as database, urogenital imaging, and urine culture Treat any underlying causes identified Initiate renoprotective therapeutic intervention$^\alpha$ if persistent renal proteinuria identified Monitor patient appropriately

(continued)

Table 3.3 (*Continued*)

Value	Interpretation	Recommendation
Azotemic dogs		
<0.4	WNRI	Review history and physical findings Perform diagnostic tests as indicated to determine source of azotemia Repeat UP:UC after treating patient for any underlying disorder identified
≥0.4	Abnormal	Review history and physical findings Perform diagnostic tests such as database, urogenital imaging, and urine culture Treat any underlying causes identified Monitor patient appropriately
≥0.5	High probability of glomerular disease	Assess patient for evidence of CKD If CKD present, treat appropriately, including glomerular renoprotective intervention[a] Monitor patient appropriately for progression of proteinuria and azotemia
≥1.0	Poor prognostic indicator for patients with CKD (increased risk of morbidity and mortality)	If initial evaluation, perform diagnostic tests to assess kidney status and overall health of patient Treat and monitor patient appropriately, including serial UP:UC determination to assess disease progression and response to therapy

Contents of table adapted from 2004 ACVIM Forum Small Animal Consensus Statement on Assessment and Management of Proteinuria in Dogs and Cats.

a = therapy such as feeding a low-protein diet and administering omega-3 fatty acid supplement and angiotensin-converting enzyme (ACE) inhibitor; patients placed on ACE inhibitors should be monitored for development of azotemia or worsening of existing azotemia.

UP:UC, urine protein to creatinine ratio; WNRI, within normal reference interval; DSCT, dipstick colorimetric test; SSA, sulfosalicylic acid turbidity test; MA, microalbuminuria test; CKD, chronic kidney disease.

MA test is reported as positive or negative, but evaluation of the depth of the associated color reaction can provide further analysis by categorizing the positive reaction as mild, moderate, or high. Some referral labs can define the extent of urine protein content to a greater degree by quantifying microalbuminuria in mg/dL. In one study microalbuminuria was detected in 19% of apparently healthy dogs and in 36% of dogs examined because of health concerns or elective procedures (Pressler et al., 2001). Two studies looking at MA in dogs predisposed to glomerulopathies appeared to support the idea that the presence of MA is a valid early marker of developing renal disease at least in the dog (Vaden et al., 2001; Lees et al., 2002). Whether the developing renal disease suggested by MA will become clinically significant is uncertain. Studies in humans (Mahmud et al., 1994; Pedersen and Milman, 1998), cats (Whittemore et al., 2007), and dogs (Whittemore et al., 2006) have suggested that MA can be associated with systemic disease. At present, the MA test is not recommended as an initial screening test for the general pet population. However, considering the results of the studies cited here, it would seem that some of the candidates likely to benefit most from MA testing would include patients with proteinuria where confirmation of the protein as albumin is desirable, as well as patients at risk for familial glomerulopathies, pets with neoplastic or chronic inflammatory disease, pets with clinical signs commonly associated with renal dysfunction, hypertensive pets, and geriatric patients. Patients positive for microalbuminuria on

Table 3.4 UP:UC interpretation and associated recommendations for feline patients with suspected or confirmed proteinuria.

Value	Interpretation	Recommendation
Nonazotemic cats		
<0.5 (noncastrated male cats may range up to 0.6)	WNRI	Monitor patient by performing DSCT, SSA, MA, and/or UP:UC every 2–4 weeks for at least two times to further define status Other diagnostic tests as indicated
0.5–1.0	Suspicious for renal proteinuria	Monitor patient by performing UP:UC periodically to confirm persistent renal proteinuria (three elevated UP:UC values found at ≥2-week intervals and not attributable to a prerenal or postrenal cause) or to identify progression Review history and physical findings Other diagnostic tests as indicated
>1.0	Abnormal	Review history and physical findings Perform diagnostic tests such as database, urogenital imaging, and urine culture Treat any underlying causes identified Monitor patient appropriately
≥2.0	High probability of glomerular proteinuria (may be tubular proteinuria [range 1–5])	Review history and physical findings Perform diagnostic tests such as database, urogenital imaging, and urine culture Treat any underlying causes identified Initiate renoprotective therapeutic intervention$^{\alpha}$, if persistent renal proteinuria identified
>5	Most commonly associated with glomerular disorders (glomerulonephritis or amyloidosis)	Review history and physical findings Perform diagnostic tests such as database, urogenital imaging, and urine culture Treat any underlying causes identified Initiate renoprotective therapeutic intervention$^{\alpha}$ if persistent renal proteinuria identified Monitor patient appropriately
Azotemic cats		
≥0.4	Abnormal	Review history and physical findings Perform diagnostic tests such as database, urogenital imaging, and urine culture Treat any underlying causes identified. In cats with CKD, initiate glomerular renoprotective intervention$^{\alpha}$ Monitor patient appropriately
≥0.43 (on initial evaluation)	Increased risk of mortality	Perform diagnostic tests to assess kidney status and overall health of patient Treat and monitor patient appropriately, including serial UP:UC determination to assess disease progression and response to therapy

Contents of table adapted from 2004 ACVIM Forum Small Animal Consensus Statement on Assessment and Management of Proteinuria in Dogs and Cats.

α = therapy such as feeding a low protein diet and administering omega-3 fatty acid supplement and angiotensin-converting enzyme (ACE) inhibitor; patients placed on ACE inhibitors should be monitored for development of azotemia or worsening of existing azotemia.

UP:UC, urine protein to creatinine ratio; WNRI, within normal reference interval; DSCT, dipstick colorimetric test; SSA, sulfosalicylic acid turbidity test; MA, microalbuminuria test; CKD, chronic kidney disease.

three or more occasions when tested at at least 2-week intervals should be considered as potentially having persistent renal proteinuria unless another source of proteinuria is obvious or identified by subsequent diagnostic procedures. Patients with persistent microalbuminuria should be monitored for progression in magnitude of proteinuria, realizing that clinically significant disease may never develop.

Although albumin is the primary protein of interest when using the methods of protein detection previously discussed, occasionally canine and feline disorders can result in increased levels of immunoglobulin in the urine. Bence-Jones proteins are free immunoglobulin light chains which are usually monoclonal and can be produced in excess by plasma cell neoplasia and some cases of B-cell lymphoma. Patients with marked hyperglobulinemia should be considered potential candidates for the presence of Bence-Jones proteins. The typical urine protein detection tests lack the sensitivity to reliably identify and/or quantify these immunoglobulin light chains. However, the SSA test can cause precipitation of Bence-Jones proteins. In the instance where the DSCT is negative for urinary protein, but the SSA test is, at least, weakly positive, Bence-Jones proteinuria should be suspected. In order to more specifically identify the presence of Bence-Jones proteins in the urine, laboratory heat precipitation or urine electrophoresis tests are needed. The heat precipitation test relies on unique characteristics of Bence-Jones proteins in regard to dissolution and precipitation at specific temperatures for identification of these immunoglobulin light chains. Electrophoresis identifies the presence of Bence-Jones proteins through the comparison of urine and serum protein peak patterns, typically documenting similar monoclonal peaks. Both the heat precipitation method and the electrophoretic method of light chain immunoglobulin identification can be difficult to interpret if concurrent albuminuria exists. It should also be noted that not all patients with disorders that produce light chain immunoglobulins will have Bence-Jones proteinuria.

Glucose

The test pad detects the presence of glucose by an enzymatic reaction involving glucose oxidase that results in a color change proportional to the amount of glucose present. When glucose is present, the color change may be associated with quantities from trace (100 mg/dL) to large ($\geq$1000 mg/dL) amounts. This reaction is specific for glucose; however enzymatic activity may be reduced in outdated test strips, resulting in false-negative results. The presence of ascorbic acid, salicylates, or tetracyclines in the urine can also lead to false-negative findings. False-positive reactions can occur in urine samples contaminated with agents such as formaldehyde, chloride, hypochlorite, and hydrogen peroxide. In addition, the enzymatic reaction may be affected by the temperature of the urine sample; thus, refrigerated samples need to be at room temperature before testing. Also, the glucose test pad on some reagent test strips (Ames) has a plastic cover over the top of the pad and urine is absorbed via the sides of the glucose test pad. Therefore, placing a drop of urine on each test pad rather than dipping the reagent strip into the urine can result in falsely decreased or negative glucose results.

Glucose passes freely into the glomerular filtrate and is reabsorbed in the proximal tubules by a sodium–glucose transport system. Glucose is not normally present in the urine in amounts that are detected by the test pad on most multiple-reagent test strips commercially available. Glucosuria occurs with any condition that causes the blood glucose concentration to rise exceeding the threshold for tubular resorption. The renal threshold for glucose reabsorption in dogs is 180–220 mg/dL and 200–280 mg/dL in cats (Feldman and Nelson, 2004). Causes of glucosuria include disorders such as diabetes mellitus, hyperadrenocorticism, acromegaly, or pheochromocytoma producing persistent hyperglycemia exceeding the renal threshold for reabsorption; conditions or situations such as stress, therapy with medications or fluids containing dextrose, pancreatitis, or meal ingestion producing transient hyperglycemia exceeding the renal threshold for reabsorption; and disorders producing proximal renal tubular dysfunction such as Fanconi syndrome, primary renal glucosuria, or renal tubular damage due to infection, hypoxia, drugs (e.g. aminoglycosides, amphotericin B), or hypercalcemia, resulting in decreased glucose absorption and subsequent glucosuria without accompanying hyperglycemia.

Ketones

Ketones are produced at low concentrations during normal lipid metabolism and excreted in undetectable amounts in the urine. The primary ketone bodies produced are acetoacetic acid, acetone, and beta-hydroxybutyrate. The DSCT detects ketones based on the reaction of acetoacetate and acetone with nitroprusside, producing an increasingly intense purple color as the ketone concentration increases. The color change from a negative reaction to a trace reaction is particularly difficult to differentiate and can be complicated by the patient's urine color, resulting in frequent false-positive results for trace readings. Although not as common, these same complicating factors can also lead to false-positive outcomes with readings in the small or moderate range. In addition, medication-related false-positive reactions can occur with drugs such as N-acetylcysteine, captopril, and penicillamine (Laffel, 1999).

The test pad is more sensitive to acetoacetic acid than acetone and does not detect beta-hydroxybutyrate, underestimating the amount of ketones present in the urine. In addition, acetoacetic acid decomposes to acetone and acetone is volatile, diffusing into the atmosphere. False-negative results or falsely decreased ketone concentrations may result from urine samples not analyzed promptly.

Ketonuria occurs when there is a shift from normal carbohydrate metabolism to lipid metabolism as the primary energy source, resulting in ketosis. Ketosis has been associated with uncontrolled or poorly controlled diabetes mellitus and conditions that result in a negative energy balance, such as starvation. A finding of ketonuria should prompt the practitioner to rule in or out diabetes mellitus as a cause by evaluating the patient for hyperglycemia and glucosuria, and the assessment of fructosamine. Because diabetic ketoacidosis (DKA) is a potentially life-threatening condition which is not always associated initially with severe clinical signs (inappetence, malaise, and vomiting), it is advantageous to identify ketosis/DKA as early as possible. Although the DSCT for ketonuria can be helpful in this identification process, this method of detection has its limitations due to lack of sensitivity to beta-hydroxybutyrate as well as the tendency for false-negatives when lower urine ketone levels are present. Alternative methods of identifying ketones include the following.

• Using the urine dipstick test pad (Multisix® Bayer Reagent Strips for Urinalysis) to test for ketonemia by using several drops of plasma obtained from a centrifuge-spun hematocrit tube. Although still subject to the test pad insensitivity to beta-hydroxybutyrate, using plasma has the potential advantages of eliminating the problem of interference with the test outcome because of strong urine color, detecting acetoacetic acid prior to reaching the renal threshold at which urine excretion occurs, and eliminating the difficulty of obtaining a urine sample from a severely dehydrated patient. One feline study indicated that the sensitivity for detection of ketones by urine reagent strips is greater for plasma samples than for urine samples (Zeugswetter and Pagitz, 2009).

- Using Acetest^{TM} (Bayer) diagnostic reagent tablets. Although this test detects the presence of ketones (acetoacetic acid, acetone) in the urine through a reaction with nitroprusside, producing a color change to give a semiquantitative result, it differs from the DSCT by incorporating lactose into the reagent tablet used to perform the test. The lactose enhances any color change associated with ketones in the sample, increasing the accuracy of interpretation. The Acetest^{TM} does not detect beta-hydroxybutyrate, but it does expand diagnostic options to some extent in that whole blood, plasma, or serum may be used as the test fluid in addition to urine. The reagent tablets should be protected from heat, moisture, and light to maintain efficacy.
- Performing measurement of urine beta-hydroxybutyrate concentration, with serum beta-hydroxybutyrate if required, on a chemistry analyzer at a reference laboratory.
- Using a portable ketonometer/glucometer (PrecisionXtra-Abbot) for in-house measurement of blood beta-hydroxybutyrate concentration (Figure 3.3). One study in cats and dogs indicated good correlation between measurements of blood beta-hydroxybutyrate concentration using a

portable ketonometer/glucometer compared to measurement by a reference laboratory chemistry analyzer (Hoenig et al., 2008). Another study indicated that measurement of blood beta-hydroxybutyrate concentration using a portable ketonometer was more accurate in predicting ketosis/DKA than measuring ketonuria by means of a DSCT (Tommaso et al., 2009).

Monitoring ketone concentrations in patients with DKA can be beneficial in evaluating efficacy of treatment. The veterinarian providing care might reasonably expect that ketone levels would decrease as DKA resolved and adjust therapy accordingly. However, urine or plasma ketone concentration monitored by the DSCT method can be misleading, keeping in mind that the ketone test pad is insensitive to beta-hydroxybutyrate and most sensitive to acetoacetic acid. As DKA starts to resolve with insulin administration and other appropriate therapy, beta-hydroxybutyrate levels drop as would be expected but acetoacetic acid levels typically increase due to the insulin-mediated conversion of beta-hydroxybutyrate to acetoacetic acid, which then acts as an energy source for peripheral tissues (Stojanovic and Ihle, 2011). Thus, ketone measurement via the DSCT can indicate that the ketotic state of the patient is not improving, or possibly worsening, despite therapy. Although the patient's clinical signs and other laboratory values should also be taken into consideration, the attending veterinarian can be misled by DSCT ketone values, particularly in the initial treatment phase of DKA, which can result in less than optimum therapeutic and monitoring decisions. Conversely, if the veterinarian is able to use one of the methods available for beta-hydroxybutyrate measurement, then ketone evaluation may be a valuable addition to the care provider's ability to assess the status of DKA patients undergoing treatment.

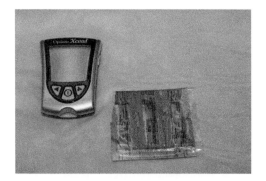

Figure 3.3 Example of portable ketonometer/glucometer which can be used for evaluation of diabetic patients.

Blood (Occult Blood, Heme)

The dipstick test pad for blood contains a peroxidase substrate which reacts with heme (iron in a porphyrin ring) molecules contained in compounds such as hemoglobin and myoglobin, and in erythrocytes. This chemical reaction results in a color change of the test pad proportionate to the amount of the heme-containing substance present.

A positive blood test pad reaction will occur with hematuria (RBCs in the urine). Erythrocytes may be present in the urine due to inflammation, trauma, neoplasia, infection, parasitism, or coagulopathy, producing a positive reaction that should correlate with microscopic visualization of RBCs in the urine sediment. Depending upon the degree of hematuria, the macroscopic appearance of the urine may or may not reflect a color change (red to brown). The urine collection process itself, especially transurethral catheterization and cystocentesis, can result in hemorrhage which will cause RBCs to appear in the urine. Consequently, the method of urine collection should always be taken into consideration as the potential cause of hematuria, particularly microscopic (urine not visibly colored red or brown) hematuria. An absence of erythrocytes in the sediment of a urine sample with a positive dipstick blood test does not rule out hematuria as the cause of the positive heme result. Lysis of RBCS may occur in urine specimens stored prior to microscopic analysis. In addition, erythrocyte lysis can occur in a urine sample which is either very alkaline (pH $\geq$ 8.0) or very dilute (USG <1.010). Although hematuria is still a likely possibility when the dipstick blood pad is positive but the urine sediment is negative for RBCs, the differential diagnoses of hemoglobinuria and myoglobinuria should still be ruled out through historical and physical findings as well as additional laboratory tests, if needed.

Unlike hematuria, which may result in lysis of RBCs in the urine with subsequent release of hemoglobin, the term hemoglobinuria is most often used to describe free hemoglobin that has spilled over into the urine from the patient's blood following an episode of intravascular hemolysis. Although both hematuria and hemoglobinuria will produce a positive reaction with the urine dipstick blood test pad and can result in a similar urine color change (usually red or brown), important distinguishing features exist (Table 3.5).

Myoglobinuria will also produce a positive reaction on the urine dipstick blood test pad. Myoglobin is a small protein released from muscle when damaged or undergoing necrosis. It easily passes into the glomerular filtrate and, when reabsorption capacity is overwhelmed, is excreted in the urine. Although damage to smooth muscle can result in the release of myoglobin, severe damage to skeletal muscle is the usual source of myoglobin in sufficient quantity to produce myoglobinuria. The resulting noncentrifuged urine sample and supernatant post-centrifugation are frequently red to brown in color. Myoglobinuria should correlate with clinical findings associated with myopathies such as muscle pain and stiffness and an increased serum creatine kinase (CK) and/or aspartate aminotransferase (AST) elevation on the patient's biochemistry profile. Other features compatible with myoglobinuria include lack of discoloration of the patient's plasma/serum, failure to visualize RBCs in the urine sediment, and, typically, absence of anemia. In some situations it may be desirable to confirm the presence of urine myoglobin through laboratory electrophoretic techniques.

When a positive reaction is obtained from the urine dipstick blood test pad, other clinical findings for the patient should always be taken into consideration when evaluating the significance of the positive result. Examining other clinical findings can not only help determine which heme-containing compound is responsible for the positive dipstick reaction but, in the case of hematuria, can also help localize the probable source of hemorrhage. Although uncommon, one

Table 3.5 Clinical features in canine and feline patients with hematuria vs. hemoglobinuria.

Feature	Hematuria patient	Hemoglobinuria patient
Urine supernatant	Clear when urine RBCs are intact; may be red (hemoglobin) to brown (oxidized hemoglobin) when urine RBCs are lysed	Often red (hemoglobin) to brown (oxidized hemoglobin)
Urine sediment	Intact RBCs visualized unless all have lysed	RBCs not visualized
Plasma or serum	Usually normal clear to straw-colored; no hemoglobinemia	Pink to red in color due to binding of hemoglobin by haptoglobin
Blood smear	No signs of hemolysis	Signs of hemolysis: RBC agglutination, spherocytes, ghost RBC and/or schistocytes
Anemia and serum/plasma total protein	Variable anemia: dependent upon cause and degree of hematuria and chronicity of blood loss Serum/plasma total protein may be within normal reference interval or may be decreased	Typically regenerative anemia Total protein usually within normal reference interval
Bilirubin	Typically no bilirubinemia or bilirubinuria	Usually bilirubinemia and bilirubinuria
Underlying cause	Multiple urogenital causes of hemorrhage: trauma, inflammation, infection, parasitism, neoplasia, iatrogenic, idiopathic, coagulopathy	Causes of intravascular hemolysis: primary (inmmune-mediated), secondary (infection, inflammation, parasites, toxins, drugs, genetic RBC defects)

consideration that should be remembered is that more than one cause of a positive dipstick heme reaction may exist in the same patient (e.g. hemoglobinuria from intravascular hemolysis and erythrocytes from hematuria). Finally, when a positive heme result does not seem to correlate with clinical findings for any particular heme-containing substance, the possibility of a false-positive reaction should be considered. In rare instances a urine sample containing bacteria or chemicals that have peroxidase activity of nonheme origin will produce a positive dipstick blood test pad reaction.

The reader is referred to Chapter 2, subheading "Color" and associated figures, for additional information on urine color variations related to heme-containing compounds and diagnosis of the causes of red or brown urine.

Bilirubin

Bilirubin is the end-product of senescent erythrocyte degradation by macrophages and the subsequent breakdown of hemoglobin, resulting in the release of unconjugated bilirubin. Unconjugated bilirubin is protein bound and cannot pass through the glomerulus and be excreted into the urine. However, after conjugation in the liver, bilirubin is water soluble and is excreted via the biliary system. Small amounts of conjugated bilirubin may then re-enter the blood and freely pass into the glomerular filtrate for excretion in urine. Bilirubin is not present normally in the urine of most domestic animals, except the dog. Due to a low renal threshold small amounts of bilirubin (trace to 1+ on the DSCT) may be detected in healthy dogs, particularly, in concentrated urine of male dogs.

Table 3.6 Guidelines for evaluation of canine and feline urine dipstick bilirubin test pad reactions. *Source:* Davies and Shell, 2002.

Bilirubin test pad reaction*	Species	Sex	Urine specific gravity	Interpretation of clinical relevance
Trace–3+	Cat	Male or female	Any	Abnormal result: pursue cause with additional diagnostic tests
Trace–1+	Dog	Male or female	≥1.020	May be seen in healthy dogs, especially male dogs: review history, physical, and lab findings
>1+	Dog	Male or female	≥1.020	Possible abnormal finding, especially in female dogs: if patient dehydrated, repeat urinalysis in rehydrated patient; in appropriately hydrated patients pursue cause with additional diagnostic tests
>1+	Dog	Male or female	<1.020	Abnormal result: pursue cause with additional diagnostic tests

*Bilirubin test pad reaction: trace, 1+ (small), 2+ (moderate), 3+ (large).

In the cat, however, the presence of bilirubin in the urine is always considered an abnormal finding and should be pursued as a sign of a potential disease process. Table 3.6 provides guidelines for interpreting the clinical relevance of bilirubinuria based on patient urine specific gravity, species, and/or sex. In both the cat and the dog bilirubinuria may precede clinical jaundice and is an early indicator of increased erythrocyte destruction (hemolytic disease), decreased bilirubin uptake or conjugation (hepatic parenchymal disorder), or decreased bilirubin excretion (cholestasis from hepatic or post-hepatic biliary dysfunction). In patients experiencing intravascular hemolysis, bilirubin may appear in the urine following absorption of free hemoglobin from glomerular filtrate by renal tubular epithelial cells with subsequent renal production and excretion of conjugated bilirubin.

The urine dipstick test pad for bilirubin is a semi-quantitative test based on an azo-coupling reaction with a diazonium salt in an acid medium. The coupling reaction produces color changes that correspond to the amount of conjugated bilirubin present. Although false-positive reactions are uncommon, pigmenturia (e.g. normal urochrome or hemoglobinuria) may obscure any color change in the bilirubin test pad and interfere with the interpretation of the dipstick reaction. It is possible to confirm the validity of a dipstick positive reaction by laboratory testing for total urine bilirubin. False-negative dipstick bilirubin reactions can occur occasionally as a result of factors related to sample handling or urine content. Bilirubin degrades in ultraviolet light and the urine sample should not be exposed to direct light. Storage of urine at room temperature can allow conjugated bilirubin to hydrolyze to unconjugated bilirubin, resulting in a lower value or negative bilirubin DSCT reaction. In some patients with bilirubinuria, bilirubin crystals may form; however, the urine dipstick bilirubin test pad may show a negative result due to putative interference with the reaction by properties of the bilirubin crystals. A false-negative reaction can also occur in a patient with a high urine concentration of ascorbic acid, which could be produced by administration of vitamin C supplementation.

4

Urine Sediment

Preparation for Microscopic Examination

Urine sediment preparations are made by placing a standard volume of 5–10 mL urine in a clean centrifuge tube and centrifuging at 165 ×G (gravitational force) or 1500 rpm for the typical urine centrifuge with a radial arm of 14.5 cm for 5 minutes. The sediment correlates to the amount of material (cells, crystals, etc.) present in the urine sample and, if present, should be visible at the bottom of the centrifuge tube. Most of the supernatant is removed (which may be used to perform urine chemistries), less 2–3 drops needed to re-suspend the sediment. Flick or gently tap the tube with a finger to remix the sediment, taking care to avoid vigorous shaking or mixing which may cause cellular artifacts and disrupt casts. With a disposable pipette, a drop of urine is transferred to a clean microscope slide and a coverslip placed over the sample. Adding 1–2 drops of a urine sediment supravital stain (Sternheimer-Malbin stain, New Methylene Blue stain) directly to the urine preparation on the microscope slide may improve the identification of cells; however, stains dilute the sample and affect the semi-quantitative evaluation of some results. Stains may also add debris, bacteria, or fungi to the sample. Urine sediment can also be examined with a Romanowski-type rapid stain such as Diff-Quik. A drop of urine sediment is placed on a clean microscope slide, smeared or rocked gently to spread the liquid, allowed to air dry,

and stained. This cytologic examination of the urine sediment will further assist in the identification of cells, bacteria, and neoplastic cells.

The microscopic examination of unstained urine sediment is performed with the microscope substage condenser lowered or with the iris diaphragm partially closed. The initial scanning of the sample is performed on low power (10× objective), allowing the examiner to evaluate the quality of preparation and the quantity of material present. Examination of the urine sediment on higher magnification (40× objective) allows the examiner to identify cells, casts, crystals, and the presence of some bacteria. The examiner may use fine focusing to assess material suspended in different planes of the fluid. The majority of microscopic findings are reported semiquantitatively as numbers per low power (10× objective) field or high power (40× objective) field on a standard amount (1 or 2 drops) of unstained urine sediment. Each finding (casts, crystals, cells) is counted by averaging the numbers counted in 10 consecutive fields. The result is reported as the average number per low power field (lpf) or high power field (hpf).

Casts

Many different types of casts (hyaline, granular, waxy, cellular, fatty, hemoglobin, mixed) can be seen in urine sediment. All casts are cylindrical molds that form in the kidney. They have a Tamm–Horsfall mucoprotein

Atlas of Canine and Feline Urinalysis, First Edition. Theresa E. Rizzi, Amy Valenciano, Mary Bowles, Rick Cowell, Ronald Tyler, and Dennis B. DeNicola.

(THM) matrix with or without cells or cellular debris and form in the lumen of the renal tubules. Tamm–Horsfall mucoprotein forms the core (matrix) of all casts and is secreted by the cells of the ascending loop of Henle, distal tubules, and collecting ducts. Casts are classified according to what, if anything, is incorporated in the mucoprotein. Decreased urine flow rate, decreased pH of urine, high solute concentration, and increased proteins (normal serum proteins or abnormal proteins) are some of the factors promoting precipitation of THM and cast formation. Each of these types of casts is briefly discussed below. In general, since casts are formed in the tubule lumen, they are much longer than they are wide but have the same diameter throughout their length and have parallel sides. Wide casts are formed in areas that have large lumens, such as the collecting ducts or dilated areas of the tubules. Thin casts are formed in narrow lumens, such as those in the loop of Henle or compressed areas of the tubules. The ends of the cast may be rounded, tapered, or straight (varies with the type of cast). Increased cast formation (cylindruria) can occur with disease in any area of the kidney (glomerulus, tubules, interstitium).

Hyaline Casts

Distinctive Features

In unstained urine, hyaline casts are pale, colorless, casts that frequently have one end that is rather blunt and rounded and another end that gradually tapers into a tail (cylindroids) (Figures 4.1–4.16). Hyaline casts have a low refractive index similar to that of urine, which makes them semitransparent. Therefore, they can be difficult to see and can easily be overlooked if the substage condenser of the microscope is not lowered. Amorphous debris frequently adheres to the outside surface of hyaline casts. One must be careful not to confuse hyaline casts with debris adhered to the surface with granular casts. Granular casts have an even distribution of material throughout the cast while hyaline casts with amorphous debris adhered to the surface have an uneven distribution of material.

Diagnostic Significance

Hyaline casts consist of THM with no cells or cellular elements as part of the cast. Low numbers of hyaline casts, less than or equal to 2 hyaline casts/lpf, can be found in concentrated urine samples from normal dogs and cats. Low to high numbers of hyaline casts may be found in urine sediment in both pathologic and physiologic disorders. Physiologically, things such as fever, strenuous exercise, diuretics, and passive congestion can cause low to high numbers of hyaline casts to be shed in the urine. Pathologically, protein-losing glomerular disease can result in low to high numbers of hyaline casts.

Next Steps

Along with good historical information and physical examination, assessment of urine and blood protein concentrations help distinguish pathologic conditions from physiologic conditions causing increased numbers of hyaline casts in the urine. Pathologic conditions are associated with a substantial increase in urine protein concentration and, possibly, a decrease in blood protein concentration, especially albumin; physiologic conditions are associated with no or only mild increases in urine protein concentration and, typically, normal blood protein concentrations.

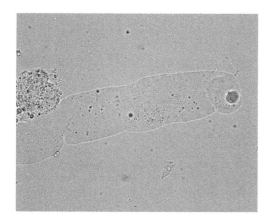

Figure 4.1 Hyaline cast (600×). The low refractive index of hyaline casts is similar to the refractive index of urine, making them difficult to see if the substage condenser of the microscope is not lowered.

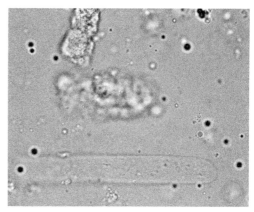

Figure 4.4 Hyaline cast with rounded end (400×).

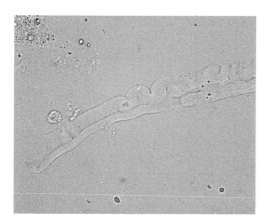

Figure 4.2 Hyaline cast (400×).

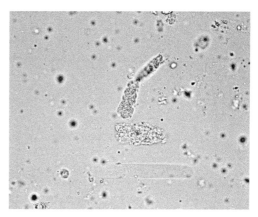

Figure 4.5 Hyaline cast (bottom) with rounded end, granular casts (middle and top).

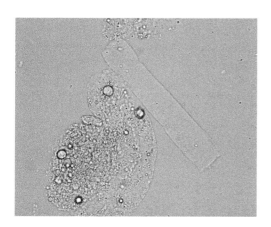

Figure 4.3 Hyaline cast with straight ends (400×).

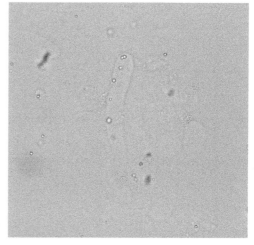

Figure 4.6 Hyaline cast (400×).

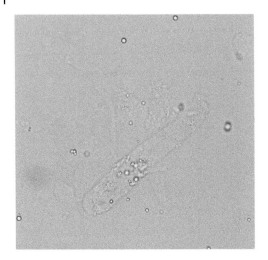

Figure 4.7 Hyaline cast with adhered lipid (400×).

Figure 4.8 Hyaline cast with rounded end (image from IDEXX SediVue Dx™ Urine Sediment Analyzer).

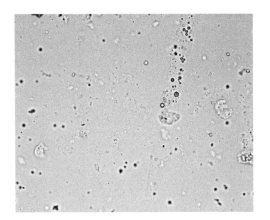

Figure 4.9 Hyaline cast with adhered lipid.

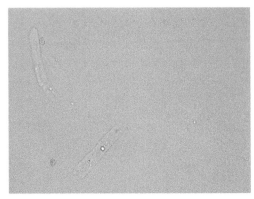

Figure 4.10 Three hyaline casts (image from IDEXX SediVue Dx™ Urine Sediment Analyzer).

Figure 4.11 Hyaline cast (image from IDEXX SediVue Dx™ Urine Sediment Analyzer).

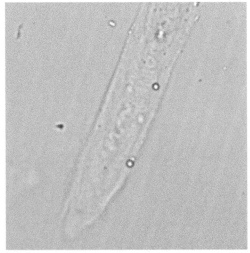

Figure 4.12 Hyaline cast (image from IDEXX SediVue Dx™ Urine Sediment Analyzer).

Figure 4.13 Hyaline cast (image from IDEXX SediVue Dx™ Urine Sediment Analyzer).

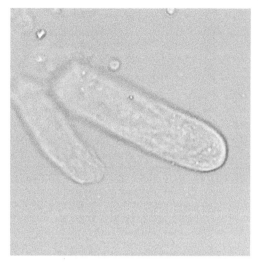

Figure 4.15 Hyaline casts (image from IDEXX SediVue Dx™ Urine Sediment Analyzer).

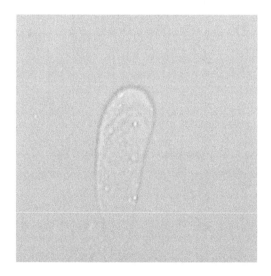

Figure 4.14 Hyaline cast (image from IDEXX SediVue Dx™ Urine Sediment Analyzer).

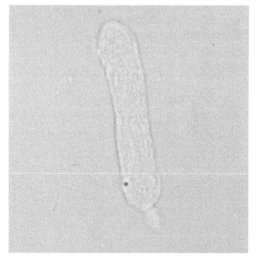

Figure 4.16 Hyaline cast (image from IDEXX SediVue Dx™ Urine Sediment Analyzer).

Cellular Casts

Distinctive Features

Cellular casts are composed of intact cells (renal tubular cells, leukocytes, erythrocytes) shed into the tubule lumen and incorporated into the THM matrix. Cellular casts are typically referred to by cell type (i.e. epithelial cell cast, white cell [leukocyte] cast, red cell [erythrocyte] cast) when only one cell type is present, or as mixed cell casts when composed of more than one cell type, or simply as cellular casts if cellular degeneration is such that the specific cell type cannot be identified. However, in some laboratories, the term cellular cast is used only to refer to a renal tubular cell cast. Cellular casts (epithelial cell, white cell, or red cell casts) may contain many cells or only a few cells caught up in a THM matrix.

Epithelial cell casts are composed of sloughed, intact renal tubular epithelial cells. They are easy to identify when cellular detail is good, as renal tubular epithelial cells are larger than leukocytes and have a large round central nucleus.

White cell casts are casts that contain a few to many leukocytes, generally neutrophils, caught up in the THM matrix. Therefore, white cell casts are basically neutrophil casts. Like epithelial cell casts, white cell casts are easy to identify when cellular detail is good, as the segmented nucleus of the neutrophil can be seen. Sometimes clumps of leukocytes are observed in urine and these should not be confused with a white cell cast.

Red cell casts are casts that contain a few to many orange to yellow looking RBCs caught up in the mucoprotein matrix (Figure 4.17). Red cell casts are very fragile and the RBCs readily disassociate causing the casts to "disappear." Therefore, fresh urine samples must be evaluated to find red cell casts.

Mixed cell casts are casts that contain more than one cell type. Mixed cell casts may contain any two or all three of the above mentioned cell types.

With all cellular casts, the cells may be very distinct if the casts are well preserved or they may show aging change (cell breakdown) and appear more like granular casts (white cell casts and epithelial cell casts) or hemoglobin casts (red cell casts). Cellular degeneration results from cellular casts remaining in the tubules and not being shed into the urine, so the degree of degeneration is a function of how long the casts have been retained in the kidney. In some cellular casts it may not be possible to determine the specific cell type due to cellular degeneration and these are typically reported as cellular casts. Also, examining urine soon after collection helps to preserve detail as casts can degenerate after collection.

Diagnostic Significance

Cellular casts are not seen in urine from normal dogs and cats and are only uncommonly seen in urine sediment from dogs and cats with renal disease. When cellular casts are observed, it is generally in association with an acute renal insult, but even then, granular casts (casts with fragmented cells) are most common, with cellular casts being a rare finding. Of the different types of cellular casts, epithelial cell casts are the most common type seen. White cell casts are rarely seen and red cell casts are very rarely seen in dog and cat urine.

Epithelial cell casts (Figures 4.18, 4.19) indicate active renal tubular necrosis or damage and suggest severe intrarenal disease. Some causes of epithelial cell casts include renal toxins, infarcts, ischemia, and acute nephritis.

White cell (leukocyte) casts are caused by intrarenal inflammation (septic or nonseptic). White cell casts generally consist primarily of neutrophils, but theoretically could include renal tubular cells or fragments of renal tubular cells. They can be seen with disorders that cause interstitial nephritis but are most commonly seen with acute bacterial pyelonephritis.

Red blood cell (erythrocyte) casts are only very rarely seen in urine from dogs and cats. They are always pathologic and indicate intrarenal hemorrhage, for example renal trauma or hemorrhagic nephritis/glomerulonephritis.

Next Steps

- Epithelial cell casts: investigate acute renal disease.
- White cell casts: investigate renal disease and consider urine culture.
- Red cell casts: investigate renal trauma or renal disease.

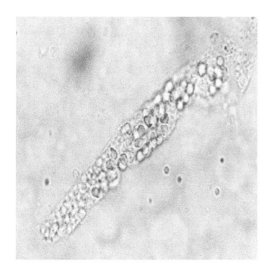

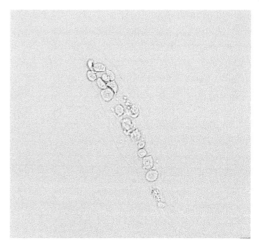

Figure 4.19 Epithelial cell cast. Intact renal tubule cells incorporated into a cast.

Figure 4.17 Red blood cell cast. These are rarely observed in urine from dogs and cats. They indicate intrarenal hemorrhage.

Figure 4.18 Epithelial cell cast. Sloughing of well-preserved renal tubular cells incorporated in a cast suggests active intrarenal disease.

Granular Casts

Distinctive Features

Granular casts (Figures 4.20–4.41) are casts that contain variably sized and shaped particulate matter (cell fragments from renal tubular cell necrosis or degeneration). These casts may be finely granular or coarsely granular. Granules may vary in size and shape within the same cast. The granules are opaque and may appear gray to yellow to black depending on their density and size. Granular casts are fragile and frequently have broken ends. Generally, coarsely granular casts are darker and shorter than finely granular casts. Like other casts, granular casts are much longer than they are wide and have parallel sides but may have an irregular or contorted shape.

Diagnostic Significance

In domestic animals, granular casts are the most common type of cast found in urine as a result of renal tubular pathology. A rare granular cast may be found in normal animals. More than one granular cast on average from 10 low power fields (10× objective) in concentrated urine is considered increased. Differentiation of finely granular and coarsely granular casts has little to no diagnostic or clinical value. Granular casts may be observed in urine sediment when: 1) a renal tubular insult lyses renal tubular cells and the cell fragments are incorporated in the mucoprotein matrix; 2) renal tubular cells are sloughed intact and incorporated in the protein matrix, forming a cellular cast but the cast is not released into the urine so the cells breakdown (aging change) and the cast becomes a granular cast before it is released; or 3) occasionally, in glomerular disease, proteins pass through the glomerulus and are incorporated in the mucoprotein matrix giving a granular appearance (glomerular disease most commonly causes hyaline casts, however). Granular casts indicate acute to recent renal damage. Infrequently, deteriorating WBC casts could resemble granular casts. WBC casts, however, are rare.

Next Steps

Investigate recent or active renal disease by reviewing patient history and physical exam findings as well as results from additional diagnostic procedures such as a complete blood count (CBC), biochemistry profile, and urinary tract imaging. Urine culture should also be considered, especially if clinical signs suggestive of infection (e.g. fever) are identified and/or stained urine sediment reveals intact WBCs or nondeteriorated WBC casts.

Figure 4.20 Granular casts (100×). These casts are composed of renal tubular cells or fragments of cells undergoing degeneration.

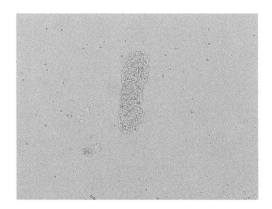

Figure 4.22 Granular cast and lipid droplets (400×).

Figure 4.21 Granular cast (200×).

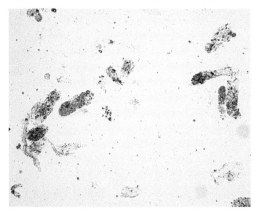

Figure 4.23 Granular casts.

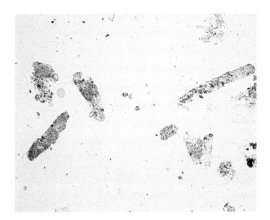

Figure 4.24 Granular casts.

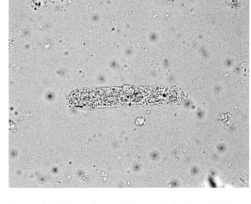

Figure 4.27 Granular cast (supravital urine stain).

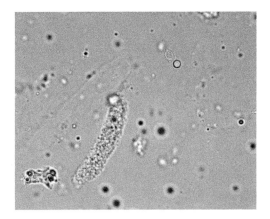

Figure 4.25 Granular cast and hyaline cast (left).

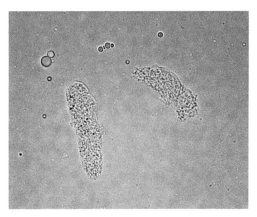

Figure 4.28 Granular cast and lipid droplets (supravital urine stain).

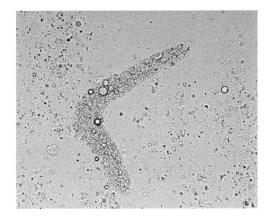

Figure 4.26 Granular cast (supravital urine stain).

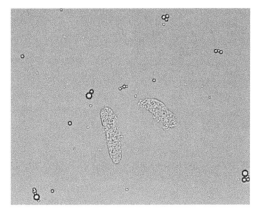

Figure 4.29 Granular cast and lipid droplets (supravital urine stain) (100×).

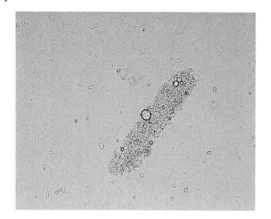

Figure 4.30 Granular cast with adhered lipid (supravital urine stain).

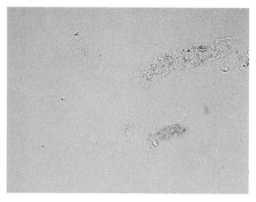

Figure 4.33 Granular cast (image from IDEXX SediVue Dx™ Urine Sediment Analyzer).

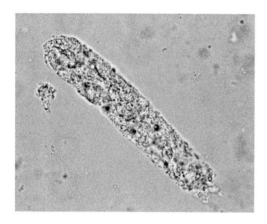

Figure 4.31 Granular cast.

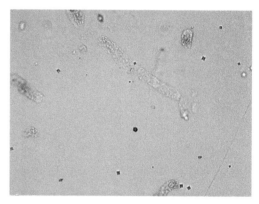

Figure 4.34 Granular cast (image from IDEXX SediVue Dx™ Urine Sediment Analyzer).

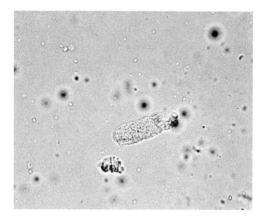

Figure 4.32 Granular cast.

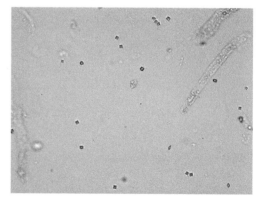

Figure 4.35 Granular cast and calcium oxalate dihydrate crystals (image from IDEXX SediVue Dx™ Urine Sediment Analyzer).

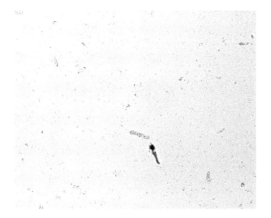

Figure 4.36 Granular cast (100×).

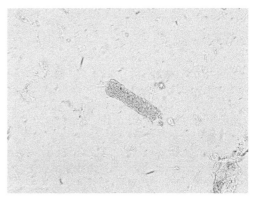

Figure 4.39 Fine granular cast.

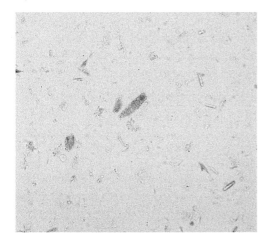

Figure 4.37 Fine granular casts.

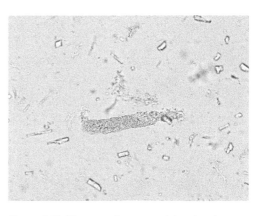

Figure 4.40 Fine granular cast and deteriorating crystals.

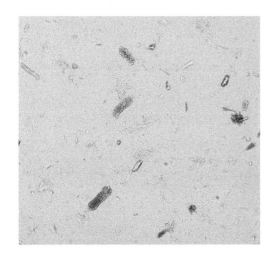

Figure 4.38 Fine granular casts.

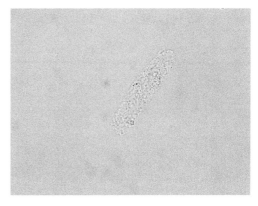

Figure 4.41 Fine granular cast.

Waxy Casts

Distinctive Features

Waxy casts (Figures 4.42–4.44) tend to have parallel sides and straight blunt ends or fractured ends. Frequently, fractures or crevices can be seen within the cast because waxy casts are very brittle. Waxy casts are easier to see in unstained urine than are hyaline casts, because they are generally thicker and denser than hyaline casts, resulting in a high refractive index. Waxy casts have a homogeneous appearance and may be colorless to gray to light yellow. They are more stable in urine than other casts.

Diagnostic Significance

Waxy casts are uncommon in urine of domestic animals. They may occur due to continued degeneration of cellular elements caught up in the THM matrix and retained in renal tubules/ducts for a prolonged period of time after an acute renal injury or in the later stages of a chronic active renal injury, and are thought to represent the end stage of granular cast degeneration. Their presence indicates damage that occurred a long time in the past and long-term nephron obstruction (intrarenal stasis) for the cast to form. Broad waxy casts (unusually wide waxy casts) indicate formation of the cast in the collecting ducts or dilated portions of the distal tubules. Since urine flow rate is normally high in this portion of the nephron and prolonged stasis of urine flow is required for waxy cast formation, high numbers of broad waxy casts suggest severe renal disease. However, the recovery phase from severe renal disease may have high numbers of broad waxy casts as nephrons shut down during oliguria are opened up as the kidney converts to a diuresis phase.

Next Steps

Investigate renal disease with special attention to long-standing renal disease.

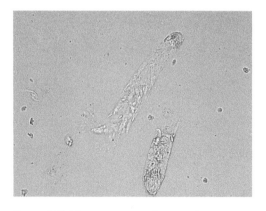

Figure 4.42 Waxy casts are easier to see in unstained urine because they appear denser and thicker than hyaline casts. Fractures can occur because waxy casts are brittle (image from IDEXX SediVue Dx™ Urine Sediment Analyzer).

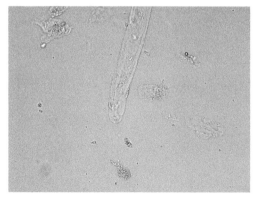

Figure 4.43 Waxy cast (image from IDEXX SediVue Dx™ Urine Sediment Analyzer).

Figure 4.44 Waxy cast (image from IDEXX SediVue Dx™ Urine Sediment Analyzer).

Fatty Casts (Lipid Casts)

Distinctive Features

Fatty casts are granular casts that contain a few to many fat droplets (oval fat bodies) (Figures 4.45–4.53). The fat droplets may vary in size from small to very large and may vary in size within the same cast. The fat droplets are refractile and may be clear to yellowish.

Diagnostic Significance

Fatty casts are seen most commonly in cats and diabetic dogs because these animals fre-quently have fatty renal tubular cells. When fatty renal tubular cells and cell fragments are incorporated in the mucoprotein matrix and degenerate, the fat from the renal tubular cell is incorporated in the cast. Therefore, fatty casts should be interpreted the same as granular casts.

Next Steps

Investigate recent or active renal disease.

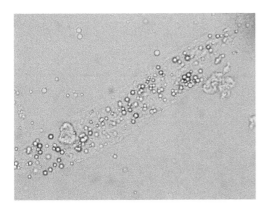

Figure 4.45 Lipid cast (600×). The fat droplets are refractile and may be clear to yellowish.

Figure 4.46 Lipid cast (100×).

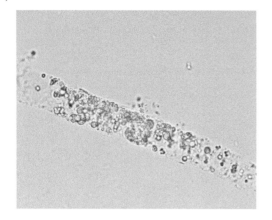

Figure 4.47 Lipid cast (500×). Fat droplets vary in size.

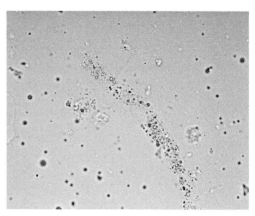

Figure 4.50 Lipid cast.

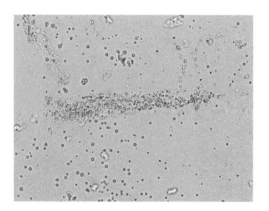

Figure 4.48 Lipid cast.

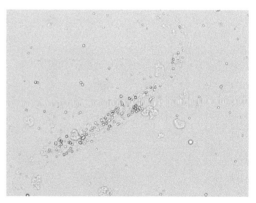

Figure 4.51 Lipid cast.

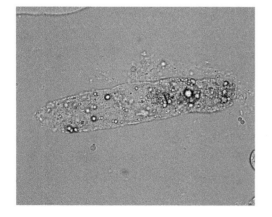

Figure 4.49 Lipid cast.

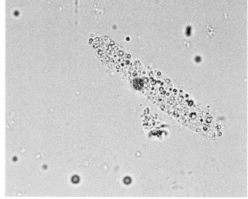

Figure 4.52 Lipid cast (supravital urine stain).

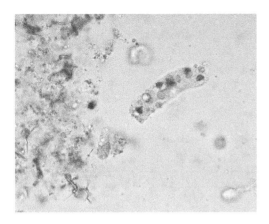

Figure 4.53 Urine from an icteric cat. Lipid cast stained with bilirubin pigment.

Hemoglobin Casts

Distinctive Features
Hemoglobin casts (Figures 4.54–4.56) are yellow to golden-brown casts with a granular texture in unstained urine.

Diagnostic Significance
Hemoglobin casts occur most commonly in association with intravascular hemolysis.

Rarely, hemoglobin casts may occur with renal hemorrhage and the subsequent breakdown of RBC casts into hemoglobin casts.

Next Steps
Investigate intravascular hemolysis (most common cause) and traumatic or hemorrhagic nephritis (less common cause and usually associated with other types of casts or evidence of renal injury or disease).

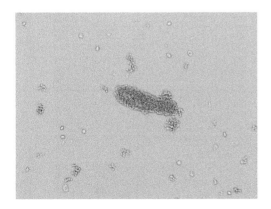

Figure 4.54 Hemoglobin cast. Urine from a dog with zinc toxicosis; these casts are most commonly associated with intravascular hemolysis.

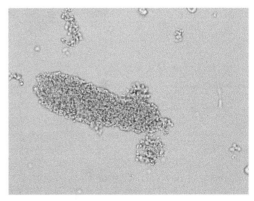

Figure 4.55 Hemoglobin cast.

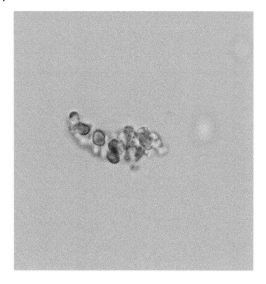

Figure 4.56 Hemoglobin cast.

Mixed Casts

Distinctive Features

Mixed casts contain components of more than one type (hyaline, granular, cellular, waxy, etc.) of cast (Figures 4.57–4.69).

Diagnostic Significance

Interpretation of mixed casts is the same as for the individual components.

Next Steps

Investigate potential causes of each of the mixed cast components.

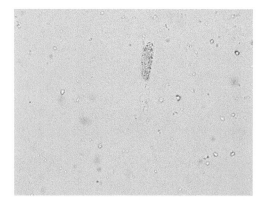

Figure 4.57 Mixed cast. The upper portion of the cast is granular and the lower portion is hyaline.

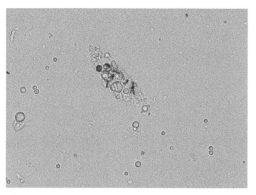

Figure 4.58 Mixed cast. Urine from an icteric cat. Bilirubin-stained renal tubule cells, lipid, and degenerating cells (granular appearance).

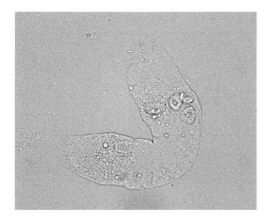

Figure 4.59 Mixed cast. A few intact renal tubular cells incorporated in the hyaline cast (1000×).

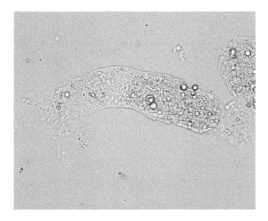

Figure 4.60 Mixed cast. Hyaline (left side) and granular (right side).

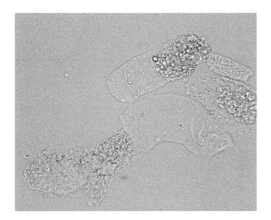

Figure 4.61 Mixed casts. Part hyaline and part granular.

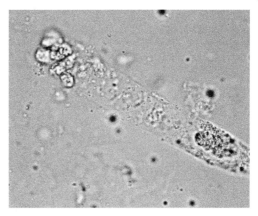

Figure 4.62 Mixed cast. The left end of the cast has intact renal tubular cells, the middle portion is hyaline and the right end of the cast appears granular.

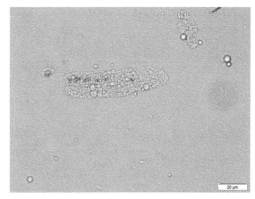

Figure 4.63 Mixed cast. Granular cast with a few lipid droplets and bilirubin crystals.

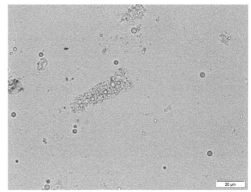

Figure 4.64 Mixed cast. Granular cast with lipid droplets.

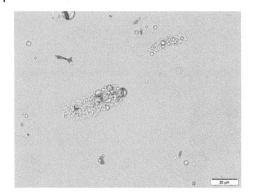

Figure 4.65 Mixed cast. Granular cast with lipid droplets and bilirubin crystals.

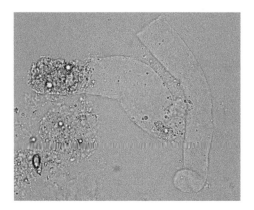

Figure 4.66 Mixed cast. The left portion of the cast is granular. The cast to the right is hyaline.

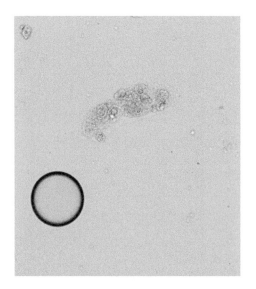

Figure 4.67 Mixed cast. Urine from an icteric cat. The renal tubular cells still have distinct margins, but are deteriorating (200×).

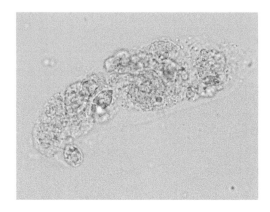

Figure 4.68 Mixed cast. The renal tubular cells are bilirubin stained (1000×).

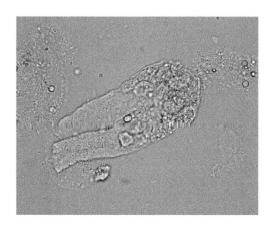

Figure 4.69 Mixed cast. Hyaline cast at both ends. The middle section contains deteriorating renal tubular cells. The cells still have distinct margins.

Pseudo Casts

Distinctive Features
Generally pseudo "false" casts lack parallel sides and other distinguishing features of true casts (Figures 4.70–4.74).

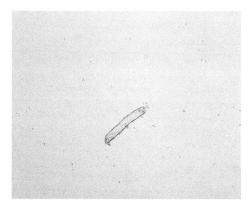

Figure 4.70 Pseudo cast. Not to be confused with true casts. These are typically mucus strands, fibers, or other contaminant.

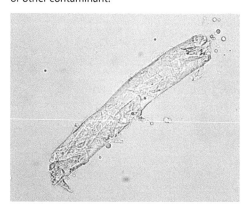

Figure 4.71 Pseudo cast.

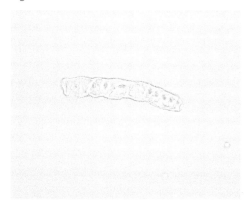

Figure 4.72 Pseudo cast (500×).

Diagnostic Significance
The main significance of pseudo casts is to not confuse them with real casts.

Next Steps
None required.

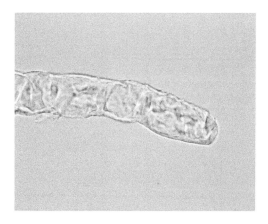

Figure 4.73 Pseudo cast (1000×).

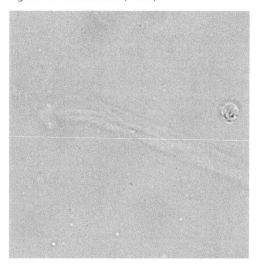

Figure 4.74 Pseudo cast (image from IDEXX SediVue Dx™ Urine Sediment Analyzer).

Crystals

A variety of physiologic and pathologic conditions can cause urine to contain crystals (crystalluria). Crystalluria depends on many factors such as urine pH, urine specific gravity, duration since urine collection, storage conditions (e.g. temperature) since collection, and the presence of inhibitors or promoters of crystal formation. Some crystals (e.g. struvite, calcium oxalate dihydrate, amorphous crystals) may be observed in urine sediment from normal animals. Other crystals are caused by or occur with inherited metabolic defects (e.g. cystine), acquired metabolic defects (e.g. ammonium urate, tyrosine), toxicities (e.g. calcium oxalate), or drug administration (e.g. sulfonamide).

Crystals Associated with Urolith Formation

Struvite/Triple Phosphate

Distinctive Features
Struvite crystals (Figure 4.75–4.112) are colorless, refractile prisms that are often "coffin lid" shaped. However, the ends may point out and occasionally they may have a fern-like appearance. Struvite crystals are composed of magnesium and ammonium phosphate. In the past, during analysis of struvite crystals, calcium was introduced and identified during the assay procedure, leading to the classification of these crystals as triple phosphate crystals (magnesium, ammonium, and calcium phosphate).

Diagnostic Significance
Struvite crystals are common findings in urine of normal dogs and cats and the most frequently identified crystal in urethral plugs of male domestic cats. Similarly, uroliths of struvite composition are among the most common uroliths occurring in the domestic dog and cat.

Next Steps
If urine struvite crystals are consistently abundant, rule out predisposing factors for struvite formation, including urinary tract bacterial infection, low urine volume, alkaline urine, and/or increased levels of dietary magnesium. Review patient history and clinical findings for any evidence of existing struvite urolith formation. Consider initiating measures to increase the patient's water intake. Feeding a diet designed for struvite dissolution or prevention may also be considered, but is generally reserved for patients with existing urolithiasis or a history of previous struvite urolith or plug formation.

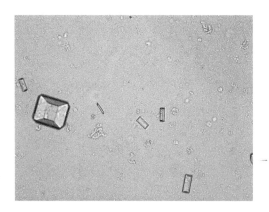

Figure 4.75 Struvite crystals (100×). They are variably sized, colorless, refractile prisms.

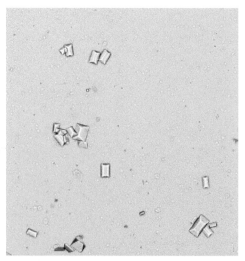

Figure 4.76 Struvite crystals (200×).

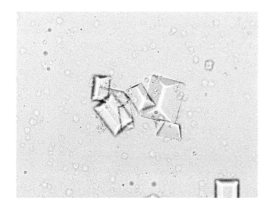

Figure 4.77 Struvite crystals, red blood cells (500×).

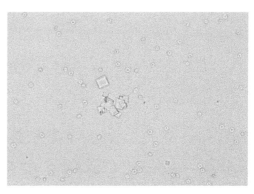

Figure 4.80 Struvite crystals and red blood cells (200×).

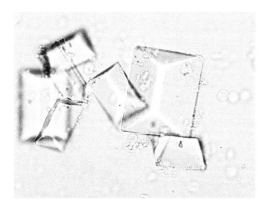

Figure 4.78 Struvite crystals (1000×).

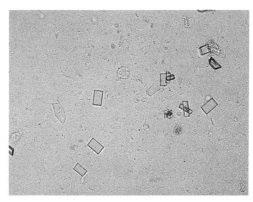

Figure 4.81 Struvite crystals and bacteria (image from IDEXX SediVue Dx™ Urine Sediment Analyzer).

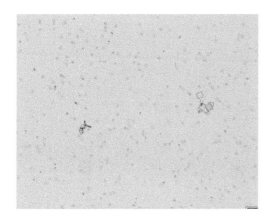

Figure 4.79 Struvite crystals and red blood cells (100×).

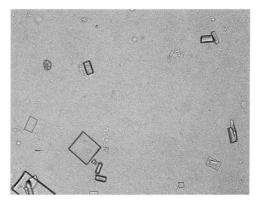

Figure 4.82 Struvite crystals and bacteria (image from IDEXX SediVue Dx™ Urine Sediment Analyzer).

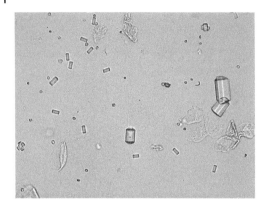

Figure 4.83 Struvite crystals and squamous epithelial cells (image from IDEXX SediVue Dx™ Urine Sediment Analyzer).

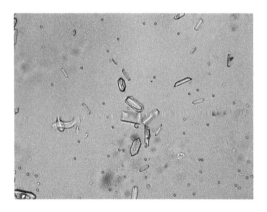

Figure 4.84 Struvite crystals and fat droplets (image from IDEXX SediVue Dx™ Urine Sediment Analyzer).

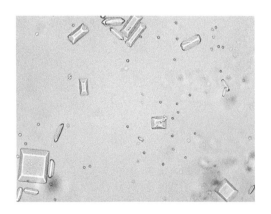

Figure 4.85 Struvite crystals and fat droplets (image from IDEXX SediVue Dx™ Urine Sediment Analyzer).

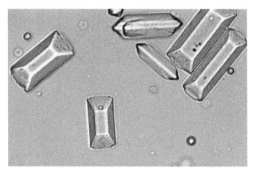

Figure 4.86 Struvite crystals (image from IDEXX SediVue Dx™ Urine Sediment Analyzer) (cropped).

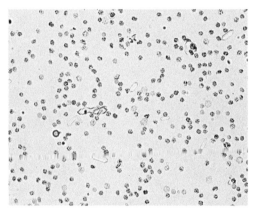

Figure 4.87 Atypical struvite and hematuria. These may be confused with calcium oxalate monohydrate crystals; however struvite crystals typically form in neutral to alkaline urine, which may help distinguish them from calcium oxalate monohydrate crystals, which form in acidic urine.

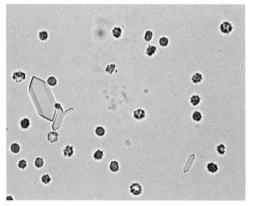

Figure 4.88 Atypical struvite and hematuria. A higher magnification inspection of these crystals reveals a prism shape (1000×).

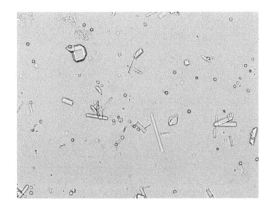

Figure 4.89 Struvite crystals.

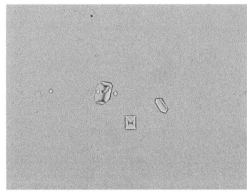

Figure 4.92 Struvite crystals, some beginning to dissolve, and background bacteria.

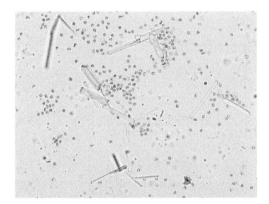

Figure 4.90 Struvite crystals and red blood cells.

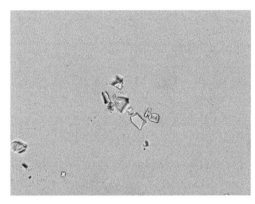

Figure 4.93 Dissolving struvite crystals and background bacteria.

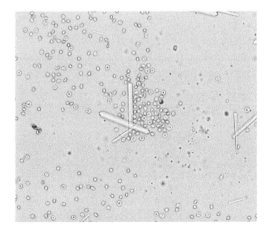

Figure 4.91 Struvite crystals and red blood cells.

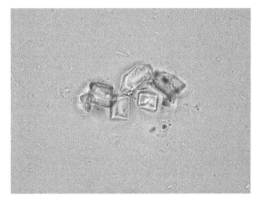

Figure 4.94 Dissolving struvite crystals and background bacteria.

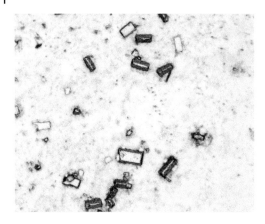

Figure 4.95 Struvite crystals (supravital urine stain; 100×). The crystals do not stain.

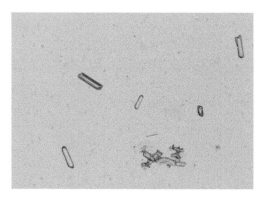

Figure 4.98 Dissolving struvite crystals.

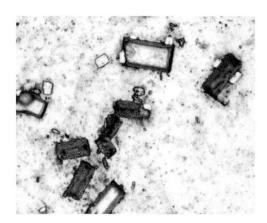

Figure 4.96 Struvite crystals beginning to deteriorate (supravital urine stain; 200×).

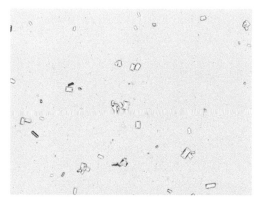

Figure 4.99 Struvite crystals and background bacteria.

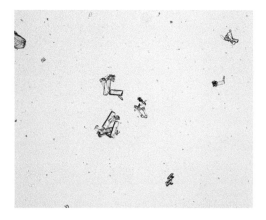

Figure 4.97 Aggregate of struvite crystals.

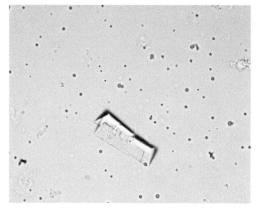

Figure 4.100 Dissolving struvite crystal (500×).

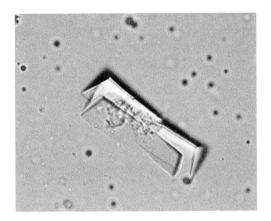

Figure 4.101 Dissolving struvite crystal (1000×).

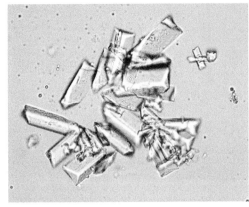

Figure 4.104 Aggregate of deteriorating struvite crystals.

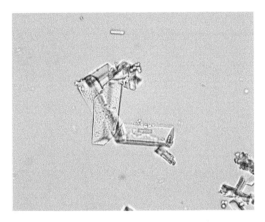

Figure 4.102 Variably sized struvite crystal aggregates.

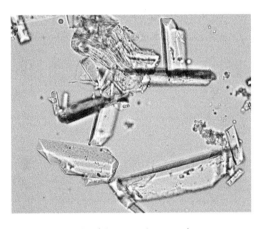

Figure 4.105 Dissolving struvite crystals.

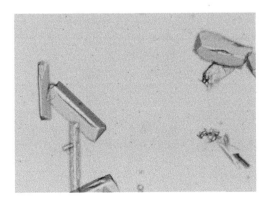

Figure 4.103 Dissolving struvite crystals.

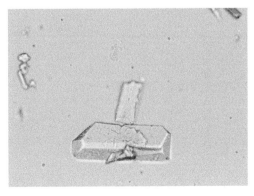

Figure 4.106 Dissolving struvite crystals.

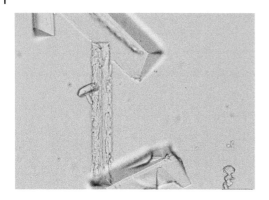

Figure 4.107 Dissolving struvite crystals.

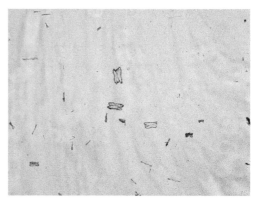

Figure 4.110 Dissolving struvite crystals.

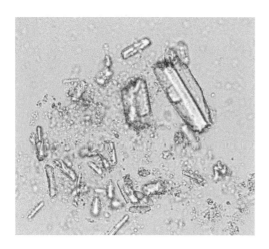

Figure 4.108 Dissolving struvite crystals.

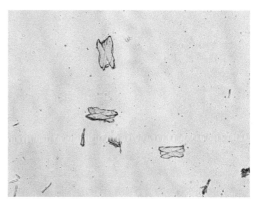

Figure 4.111 Dissolving struvite crystals.

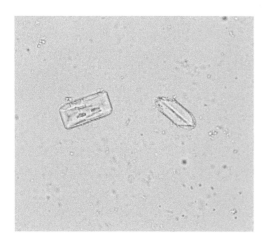

Figure 4.109 Dissolving struvite crystals.

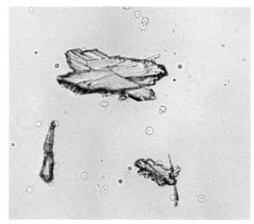

Figure 4.112 Dissolving struvite crystals.

Calcium Oxalate Dihydrate

Distinctive Features

Calcium oxalate dihydrate crystals (Figures 4.113–4.127) are colorless octahedrals that appear square to slightly rectangular with a "Maltese cross" (an "X" connecting the four corners). Occasionally these crystals may take on a cube-like form. Calcium oxalate dihydrate crystals can vary tremendously in size, ranging from so small they are barely discernible to very large. However, upon focusing up and down the "Maltese cross" can be discerned, identifying them as calcium oxalate dihydrate crystals.

Diagnostic Significance

Occasionally, normal animals may have a few calcium oxalate dihydrate crystals in their urine sediment. Ingestion of oxalate-containing diets (e.g. certain plants) enhances their production. Identification of moderate to abundant numbers of calcium oxalate dihydrate crystals in urine from dogs and cats suggests ethylene glycol ingestion. However, calcium oxalate dihydrate crystals *are* *not* pathognomonic for ethylene glycol ingestion. Urine sediment does not contain calcium oxalate dihydrate crystals in some cases of ethylene glycol toxicity. Calcium oxalate dihydrate crystals may also contribute to the formation of calcium oxalate uroliths, which are frequently found in dogs and cats.

Next Steps

Review history, clinical findings, and clinical chemistry results for evidence of ethylene glycol toxicity and the possible presence of calcium oxalate uroliths. The persistent presence of calcium oxalate dihydrate crystals in the urine without evidence of ethylene glycol toxicity may warrant checking for other predisposing causes of calcium oxalate formation, including hypercalcemia, hypercalciuria, increased dietary oxalates, and acidic urine. Calcium oxalate dihydrate crystalluria may indicate the need to increase the patient's water consumption. Feeding a diet compatible with calcium oxalate prevention is also an option, but is most commonly recommended for patients with a history of previous calcium oxalate urolith formation.

Figure 4.113 Calcium oxalate dihydrate crystals are colorless and octahedral (200×).

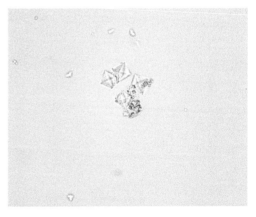

Figure 4.114 Calcium oxalate dihydrate crystals (400×).

Figure 4.115 Calcium oxalate dihydrate crystals (100×).

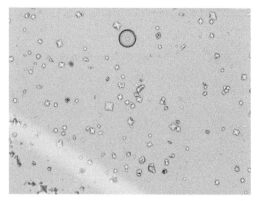

Figure 4.118 Calcium oxalate dihydrate crystals of varying sizes (200×).

Figure 4.116 Calcium oxalate dihydrate crystals (400×).

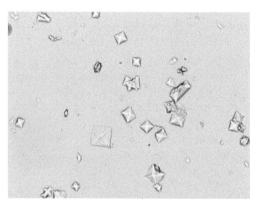

Figure 4.119 Calcium oxalate dihydrate crystals (500×).

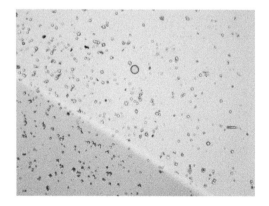

Figure 4.117 Calcium oxalate dihydrate crystals of varying sizes (100×).

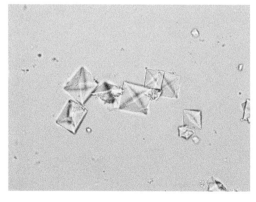

Figure 4.120 Calcium oxalate dihydrate crystals (1000×).

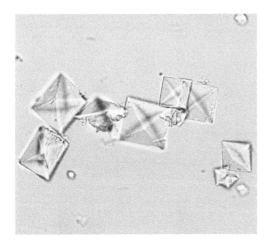

Figure 4.121 Calcium oxalate dihydrate crystals.

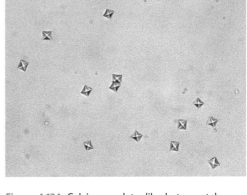

Figure 4.124 Calcium oxalate dihydrate crystals (image from IDEXX SediVue Dx™ Urine Sediment Analyzer")

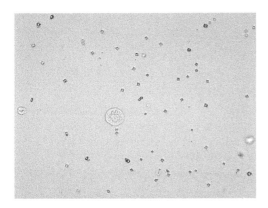

Figure 4.122 Calcium oxalate dihydrate crystals (image from IDEXX SediVue Dx™ Urine Sediment Analyzer).

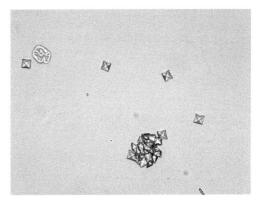

Figure 4.125 Aggregate and individual calcium oxalate dihydrate crystals (image from IDEXX SediVue Dx™ Urine Sediment Analyzer).

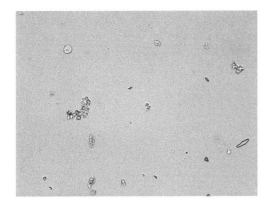

Figure 4.123 Calcium oxalate dihydrate crystals (image from IDEXX SediVue Dx™ Urine Sediment Analyzer).

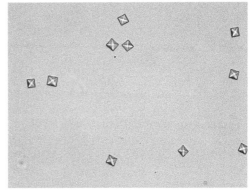

Figure 4.126 Calcium oxalate dihydrate crystals (image from IDEXX SediVue Dx™ Urine Sediment Analyzer).

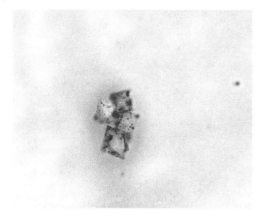

Figure 4.127 Calcium oxalate dihydrate crystals do not stain with supravital urine stain, but adhered particulate matter can stain giving the appearance of stained crystals (1000×).

Calcium Oxalate Monohydrate

Distinctive Features

Calcium oxalate monohydrate crystals vary in size. They may be elongated, flat, translucent crystals that come to a point at both ends (picket fence-like) (Figures 4.128–4.138) appearing similar to hippuric acid crystals, or they may be spindle, oval (hemp seed) (Figures 4.139–4.146), barrel (Figures 4.147, 4.148), or dumbbell shaped (Figures 4.149–4.157). Calcium oxalate monohydrate crystals are the most common type of calcium oxalate crystal seen during ethylene glycol intoxication.

Diagnostic Significance

When calcium oxalate monohydrate crystals are identified in urine from dogs and cats, ethylene glycol ingestion should be suspected and investigated. However, urine sediment does not contain calcium oxalate monohydrate crystals in some cases of ethylene glycol toxicity. Calcium oxalate monohydrate crystals can also be involved in the formation of calcium oxalate uroliths.

Next Steps

Review history, clinical findings, and clinical chemistry results for evidence of ethylene glycol toxicity or the presence of calcium oxalate uroliths. Calcium oxalate monohydrate crystals are infrequently found in normal animals, even with ingestion of oxalate-containing diets or plants; therefore, ethylene glycol ingestion should be considered and investigated when calcium oxalate monohydrate crystals are observed. In the absence of evidence of ethylene glycol toxicity, the presence of calcium oxalate monohydrate crystalluria should prompt a search for predisposing causes of calcium oxalate formation, including not only dietary sources of oxalate but also hypercalcemia, hypercalciuria, and acidic urine. Therapeutically, increasing patient water consumption should be considered. Feeding a diet compatible with calcium oxalate prevention can be considered but is generally reserved for patients with a history of previous calcium oxalate urolith formation.

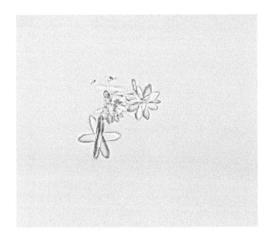

Figure 4.128 An aggregate of calcium oxalate monohydrate crystals in the urine of a dog with ethylene glycol toxicosis (200×).

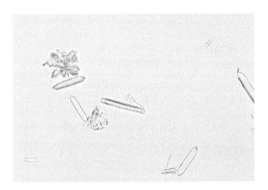

Figure 4.129 Calcium oxalate monohydrate crystals (200×). They are elongated and flat with a point at both ends (picket fence-like).

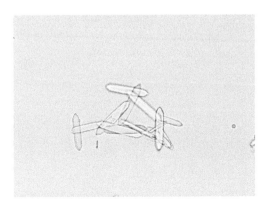

Figure 4.130 Calcium oxalate monohydrate crystals (200×).

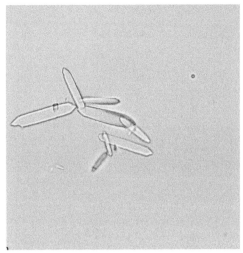

Figure 4.131 Calcium oxalate monohydrate crystals (500×).

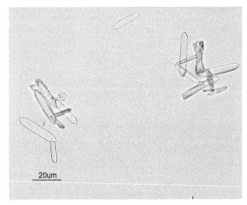

Figure 4.132 Calcium oxalate monohydrate crystals.

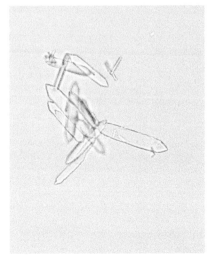

Figure 4.133 Calcium oxalate monohydrate crystals.

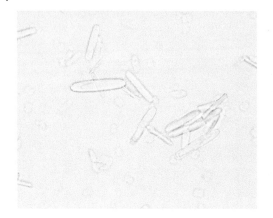

Figure 4.134 Calcium oxalate monohydrate crystals (1000×).

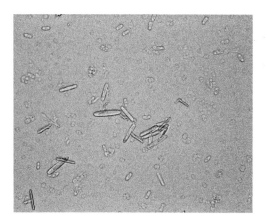

Figure 4.135 Calcium oxalate monohydrate crystals (supravital urine stain; 100×). The crystals do not stain with supravital urine stains.

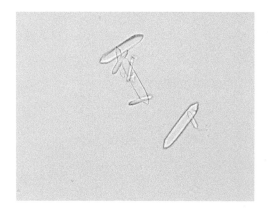

Figure 4.136 Calcium oxalate monohydrate crystals.

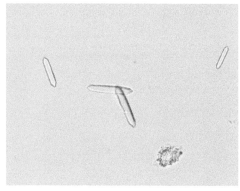

Figure 4.137 Calcium oxalate monohydrate crystals.

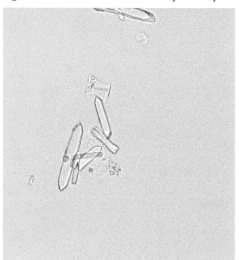

Figure 4.138 Calcium oxalate monohydrate crystals.

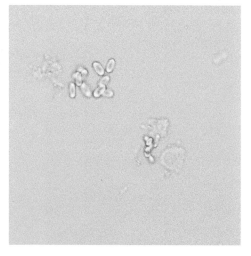

Figure 4.139 Calcium oxalate monohydrate crystals: oval or "hemp seed" appearance. Urine from a dog with calcium oxalate uroliths.

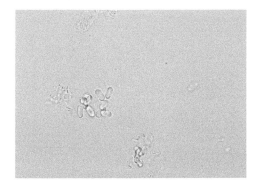

Figure 4.140 Calcium oxalate monohydrate crystals: oval or "hemp seed" appearance.

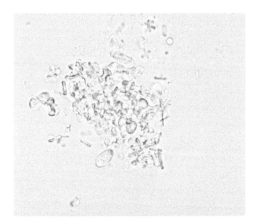

Figure 4.141 Aggregate of calcium oxalate monohydrate crystals: oval or "hemp seed" and "barbell" appearance. Urine from a dog with calcium oxalate uroliths.

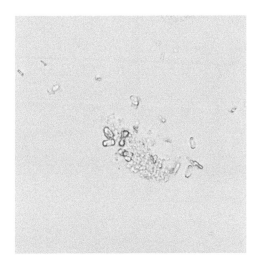

Figure 4.142 Calcium oxalate monohydrate crystals: oval or "hemp seed" and "barbell" appearance.

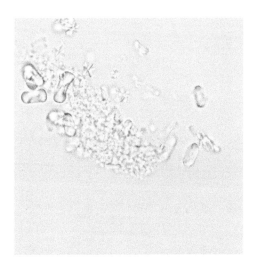

Figure 4.143 Calcium oxalate monohydrate crystals: oval or "hemp seed" and "barbell" appearance.

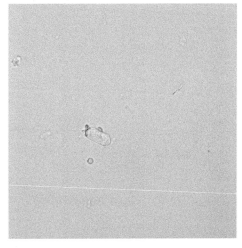

Figure 4.144 Calcium oxalate monohydrate crystal: oval or "hemp seed" appearance.

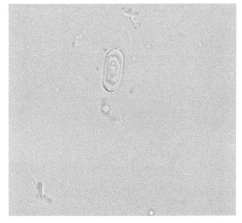

Figure 4.145 Calcium oxalate monohydrate crystal: oval or "hemp seed" appearance.

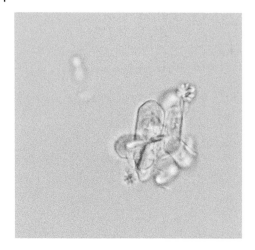

Figure 4.146 Aggregate of calcium oxalate monohydrate crystals: oval or "hemp seed" appearance.

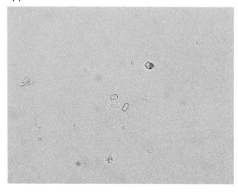

Figure 4.147 Calcium oxalate monohydrate crystals: oval or "barrel shape" appearance.

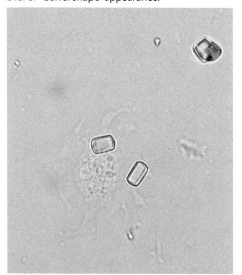

Figure 4.148 Calcium oxalate monohydrate crystals: oval or "barrel shape" appearance (1000×).

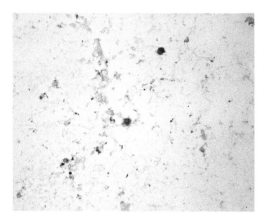

Figure 4.149 Urine from a dog. Calcium oxalate monohydrate crystals: dumbbell-shape (supravital urine stain; 200×). The crystals will not stain with supravital urine stain.

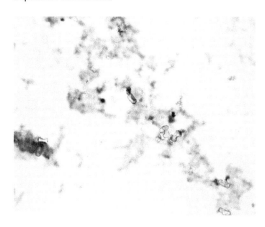

Figure 4.150 Calcium oxalate monohydrate crystals: dumbbell shape (supravital urine stain; 500×).

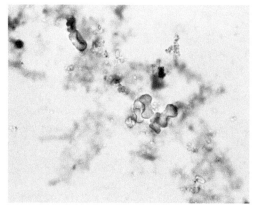

Figure 4.151 Calcium oxalate monohydrate crystals: dumbbell shape (supravital urine stain; 1000×).

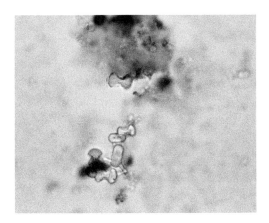

Figure 4.152 Calcium oxalate monohydrate crystals: dumbbell shape (supravital urine stain; 1000×).

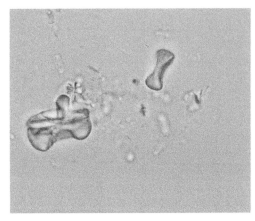

Figure 4.155 Calcium oxalate monohydrate crystals: dumbbell shape (1000×).

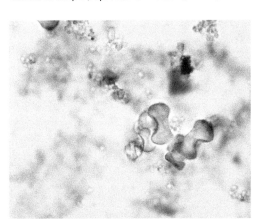

Figure 4.153 Calcium oxalate monohydrate crystals: dumbbell shape (supravital urine stain; 1000×).

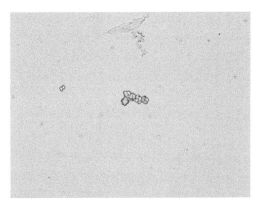

Figure 4.156 Aggregate of calcium oxalate monohydrate crystals: dumbbell shape and calcium oxalate dihydrate (left side) (100×).

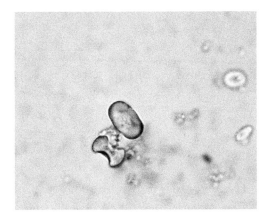

Figure 4.154 Calcium oxalate monohydrate crystals: dumbbell shape and hemp seed shape (supravital urine stain; 1000×).

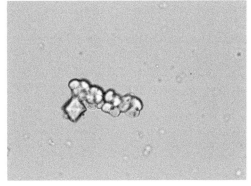

Figure 4.157 Calcium oxalate monohydrate crystals (dumbbell shape) and calcium oxalate dihydrate (600×).

Calcium Phosphate

Distinctive Features
Calcium phosphate crystals (Figures 4.158–4.166) may occur as colorless plates or needles. The plates are thin and flat, while the needles are long and thin.

Diagnostic Significance
Calcium phosphate crystals can be seen in association with conditions promoting hypercalciuria and/or hyperphosphaturia. Rarely, calcium phosphate uroliths may occur in the dog or cat.

Next Steps
Review the patient's history, clinical findings, and biochemical profile for evidence of conditions contributing to hypercalciuria and hyperphosphaturia. In the dog, such conditions include hyperparathyroidism, hyperadrenocorticism, idiopathic hypercalciuria, and distal renal tubular acidosis. Calcium phosphate urolith formation, especially nephroliths, should also be investigated. Increasing patient water consumption should be considered in patients with persistent calcium phosphate crystalluria or uroliths. Eliminating or limiting administration of medications enhancing calcium excretion (e.g. furosemide, glucocorticoids, and drugs with increased sodium content) may be advisable. High-fiber diets may be beneficial in reduction of urinary calcium excretion, and diets with high sodium content should be avoided.

Figure 4.158 Urine from a dog. Calcium phosphate (500×) crystals are colorless plates or needles.

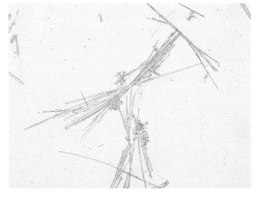

Figure 4.160 Urine from a dog. Calcium phosphate crystals (200×).

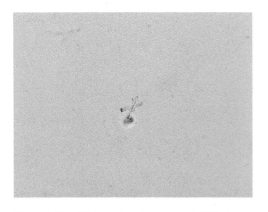

Figure 4.159 Calcium phosphate crystals (500×).

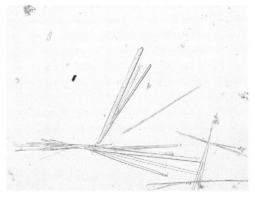

Figure 4.161 Calcium phosphate crystals (200×).

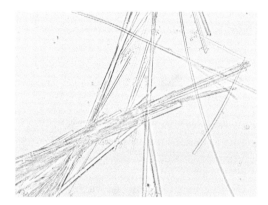

Figure 4.162 Calcium phosphate crystals (500×).

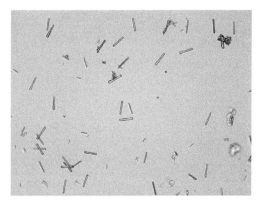

Figure 4.165 Calcium phosphate crystals (image from IDEXX SediVue Dx™ Urine Sediment Analyzer).

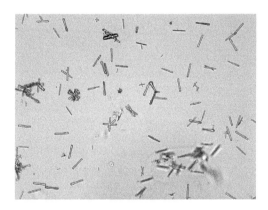

Figure 4.163 Calcium phosphate crystals (image from IDEXX SediVue Dx™ Urine Sediment Analyzer).

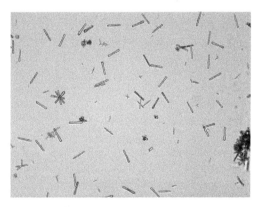

Figure 4.166 Calcium phosphate crystals (image from IDEXX SediVue Dx™ Urine Sediment Analyzer).

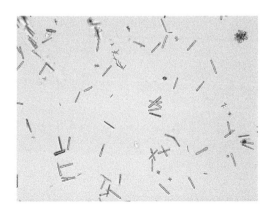

Figure 4.164 Calcium phosphate crystals (image from IDEXX SediVue Dx™ Urine Sediment Analyzer).

Urate/Ammonium Biurate

Distinctive Features

Urate (ammonium urate) crystals (also called ammonium biurate crystals) are usually brown or yellow–brown spheres with long, irregular protrusions (thorn apple appearance) (Figures 4.167–4.184), but they can also appear as a brown to yellow–brown smooth-surface spheres with internal radiating striations (Figures 4.185–4.193). The smooth surface ammonium urate crystals may be confused with calcium carbonate crystals, which are common in equine urine samples, but are not found in canine or feline urine.

Diagnostic Significance

Ammonium urate crystals rarely occur in urine from healthy dogs and cats with the exception of Dalmatians and English bulldogs. In cats and dog breeds other than Dalmatians and English bulldogs, moderate or large numbers of urate crystals suggest high blood ammonia or uric acid levels due, most commonly, to a portal vascular anomaly; they may also be seen in urine from dogs and cats with urate uroliths caused by disorders other than portal vascular anomalies. It should be noted that ammonium urate crystals are not always present in all portal vascular anomalies.

Next Steps

For Damations and English bulldogs, urate crystalluria does not necessitate further investigation (unless clinical signs or other evidence suggests a disorder such as gout, portal vascular anomaly, or the presence of uroliths).

For other dog breeds and cats, history (including review of the patient's diet), clinical findings, and clinical laboratory results should be examined for evidence of hepatic dysfunction, especially portal vascular anomaly, or urolithiasis. It should be remembered that urate urolithiasis formation in cats is frequently idiopathic. Additional diagnostic procedures, such as radiographs, should be performed as indicated by findings from this work-up.

Therapeutically, persistent urate crystalluria may indicate the need to implement procedures to increase patient water consumption. Feeding a diet compatible with urate dissolution or prevention could be considered, but is most commonly recommended for patients with existing urolithiasis or a history of urate urolith formation. If an underlying cause, such as portal vascular anomaly, has been identified in the diagnostic work-up, therapeutic measures appropriate for the identified disorder should be considered.

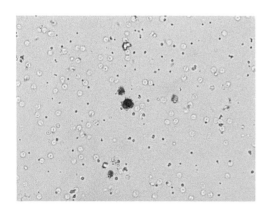

Figure 4.167 Urine from a dog. Ammonium urate crystals are usually brown or yellow–brown spheres with irregular surface protrusions (thorn apple appearance). Red blood cells in the background (50×).

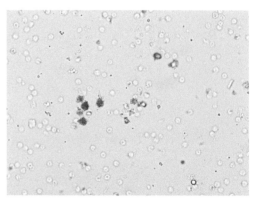

Figure 4.168 Ammonium urate crystals, numerous red blood cells and a single calcium oxalate dihydrate crystal (center) (500×).

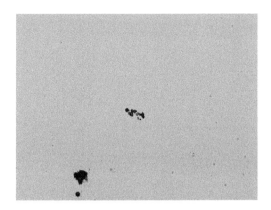

Figure 4.169 Ammonium urate crystals can vary in size (200×).

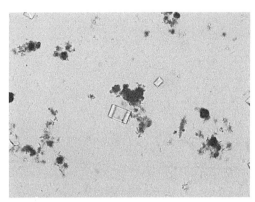

Figure 4.172 Ammonium urate crystals, struvite crystals, and bacteria (400×).

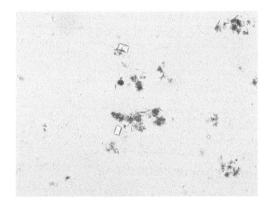

Figure 4.170 Ammonium urate crystals, two struvite crystals, and bacteria (400×).

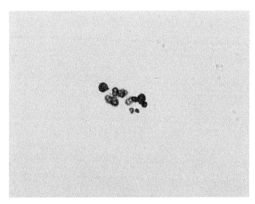

Figure 4.173 Ammonium urate crystals (400×).

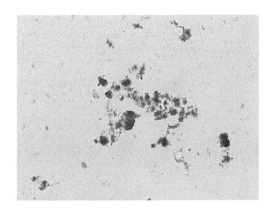

Figure 4.171 Ammonium urate crystals and bacteria (400×).

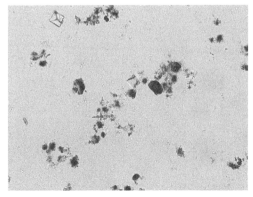

Figure 4.174 Ammonium urate crystals, struvite crystals, and bacteria (400×).

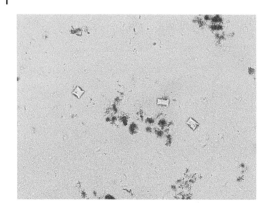

Figure 4.175 Ammonium urate crystals, struvite crystals, and bacteria (400×).

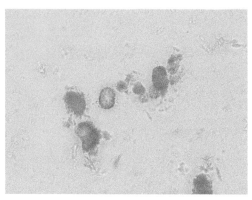

Figure 4.178 Ammonium urate crystals (1000×).

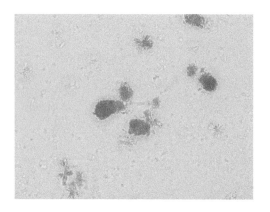

Figure 4.176 Ammonium urate crystals and bacteria (400×).

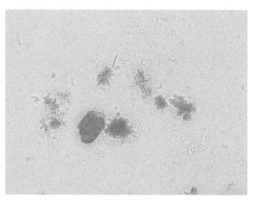

Figure 4.179 Ammonium urate crystals (1000×).

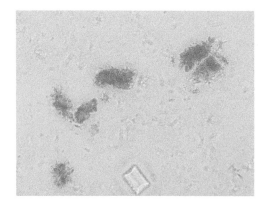

Figure 4.177 Ammonium urate crystals, bacteria, and struvite crystal (1000×).

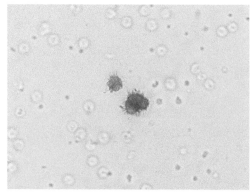

Figure 4.180 Ammonium urate crystals and RBCs (1000×).

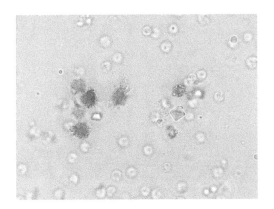

Figure 4.181 Ammonium urate crystals, calcium oxalate dihydrate, and red blood cells (1000×).

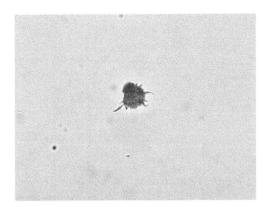

Figure 4.182 Ammonium urate crystal (1000×).

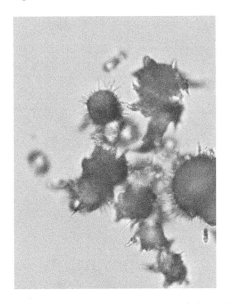

Figure 4.183 Ammonium urate crystals (1000×).

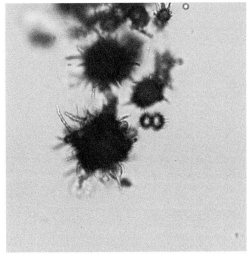

Figure 4.184 Ammonium urate crystals (1000×).

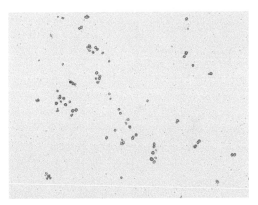

Figure 4.185 Ammonium urate crystals may have a smooth surface (100×).

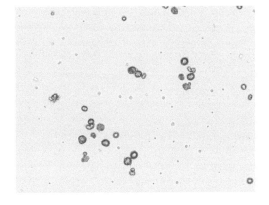

Figure 4.186 Ammonium urate crystals (200×).

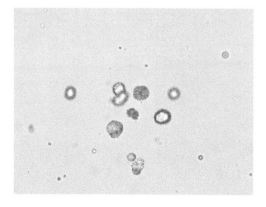

Figure 4.187 Ammonium urate crystals (200×).

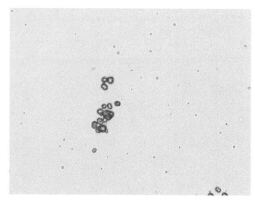

Figure 4.190 Ammonium urate crystals (100×).

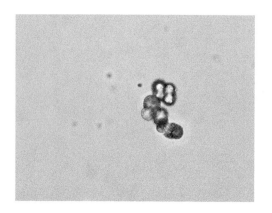

Figure 4.188 Ammonium urate crystals (500×).

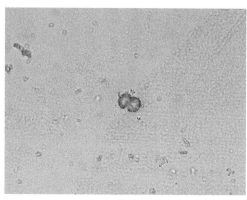

Figure 4.191 Ammonium urate crystals (500×).

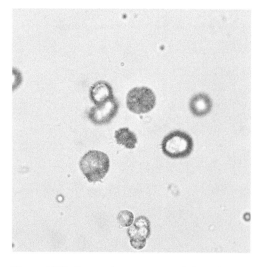

Figure 4.189 Ammonium urate crystals (500×).

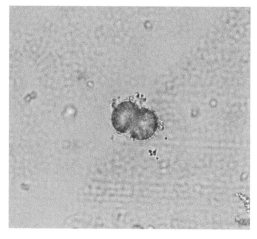

Figure 4.192 Ammonium urate crystals (1000×).

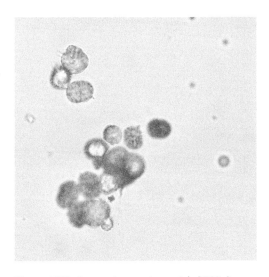

Figure 4.193 Ammonium urate crystals (1000×).

Uric Acid

Distinctive Features
Uric acid crystals (Figures 4.194–4.205) are usually yellow or yellow–brown, diamond or rhomboidal plates that sometimes contain concentric rings. Rosettes containing aggregates of many uric acid crystals sometimes develop. Occasionally, uric acid crystals are six-sided and resemble cystine crystals. How-ever, the presence of the typical diamond or rhomboid forms allows these six-sided crystals to be recognized as uric acid crystals.

Diagnostic Significance
Same as for ammonium urate crystals.

Next Steps
Same as for ammonium urate crystals.

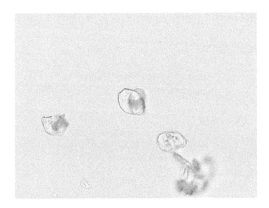

Figure 4.194 Uric acid crystals in urine from a cat. Uric acid crystals are usually yellow or yellow–brown, diamond or rhomboid plates with occasional concentric rings (500×).

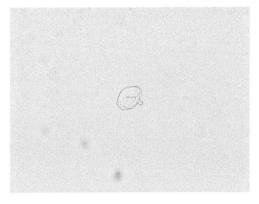

Figure 4.195 Uric acid crystal (500×).

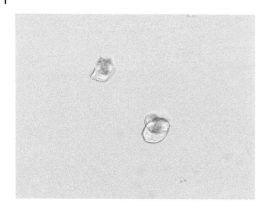

Figure 4.196 Uric acid crystals (500×).

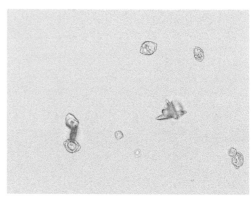

Figure 4.199 Uric acid crystals (500×).

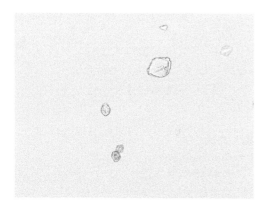

Figure 4.197 Uric acid crystals in urine from a dog (500×).

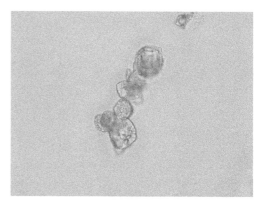

Figure 4.200 Uric acid crystals (1000×).

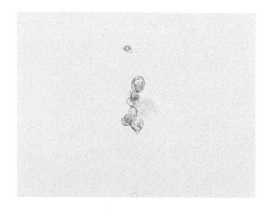

Figure 4.198 Uric acid crystals (500×).

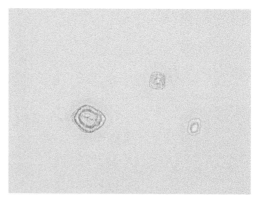

Figure 4.201 Uric acid crystals (1000×).

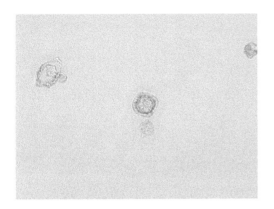

Figure 4.202 Uric acid crystals (1000×).

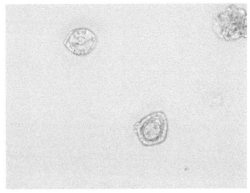

Figure 4.204 Uric acid crystals (1000×).

Figure 4.203 Uric acid crystal (1000×).

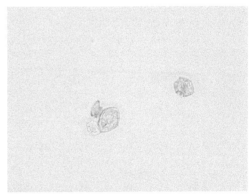

Figure 4.205 Uric acid crystals (1000×).

Cystine

Distinctive Features

Cystine crystals (Figures 4.206–4.237) are colorless, flat, and hexagonal. The sides may or may not be of equal length and the crystals may appear layered. They are best observed with reduced lighting.

Diagnostic Significance

Cystine crystalluria is never considered a normal finding and suggests an inherited defect in cystine metabolism that may lead to development of cystine uroliths. Acidic urine is a contributory factor to crystal and urolith formation. Cystine uroliths are uncommon occurrences in both dogs and cats.

Next Steps

Establish persistence of cystinuria through repeat urinalysis, using a fresh, nonrefrigerated urine sample. Monitor for development of cystine uroliths. Increasing patient water consumption should be considered. Initiation of diets compatible with cystine urolith prevention (dogs and cats) or dissolution (dogs) is generally reserved for patients with existing uroliths or a history of previous cystine urolith formation. Screening should be considered (PennGen) to identify genetic characteristics and, in the case of the affected intact, male dog, to help determine if castration may be beneficial to reduce cystine urine excretion, in addition to preventing transmission of this genetic disorder.

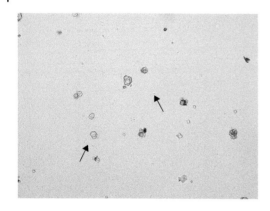

Figure 4.206 Urine from a dog. Cystine crystals and calcium oxalate dihydrate, rare sperm (arrows) (200×).

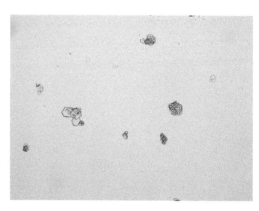

Figure 4.209 Aggregates of cystine crystals, calcium oxalate dihydrate crystals, rare sperm (200×).

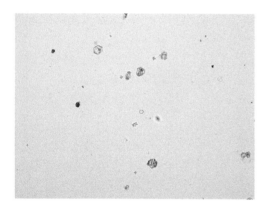

Figure 4.207 Cystine crystals and calcium oxalate dihydrate (200×).

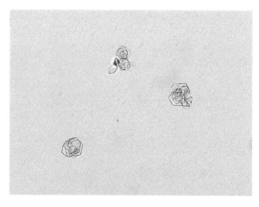

Figure 4.210 Aggregates of cystine crystals (500×).

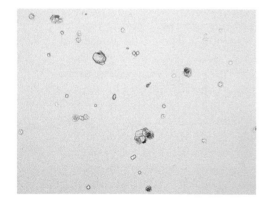

Figure 4.208 Aggregates of cystine crystals and calcium oxalate dihydrate crystals (200×).

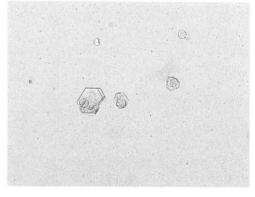

Figure 4.211 Aggregates of cystine crystals, one calcium oxalate dihydrate crystal, and sperm (500×).

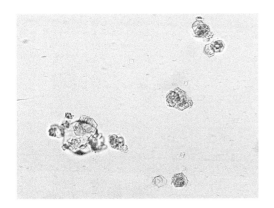

Figure 4.212 Aggregates of cystine crystals and calcium oxalate dihydrate crystals (500×).

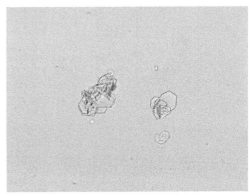

Figure 4.215 Aggregates of cystine crystals (1000×).

Figure 4.213 Cystine crystals (500×).

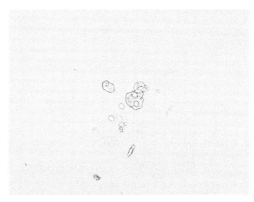

Figure 4.216 Cystine crystals (500×).

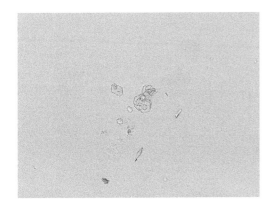

Figure 4.214 Cystine crystals (500×).

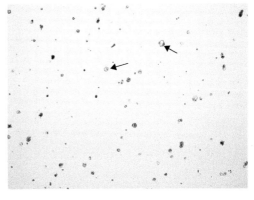

Figure 4.217 Cystine crystals (arrows) (100×).

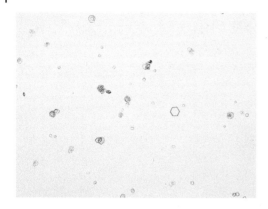

Figure 4.218 Cystine crystals, calcium oxalate dihydrate (200×).

Figure 4.221 Aggregate of cystine crystals, calcium oxalate dihydrate, sperm (500×).

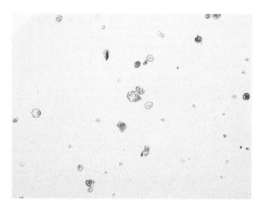

Figure 4.219 Cystine crystals, calcium oxalate dihydrate (200×).

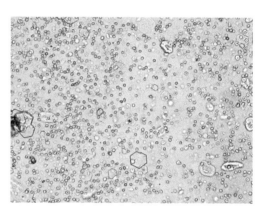

Figure 4.222 Cystine crystals, red blood cells, and squamous cells (image from IDEXX SediVue Dx™ Urine Sediment Analyzer).

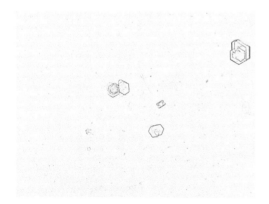

Figure 4.220 Cystine crystals, calcium oxalate dihydrate, sperm (500×).

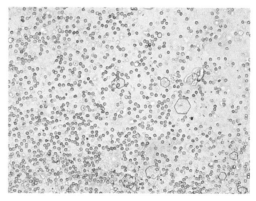

Figure 4.223 Cystine crystals and red blood cells (image from IDEXX SediVue Dx™ Urine Sediment Analyzer).

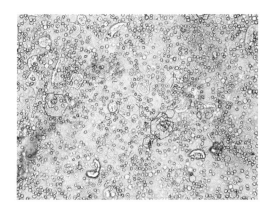

Figure 4.224 Cystine crystals, red blood cells, and squamous cells (image from IDEXX SediVue Dx™ Urine Sediment Analyzer).

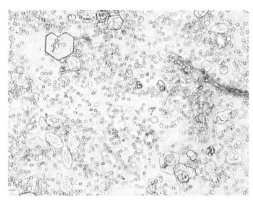

Figure 4.227 Cystine crystals, red blood cells, and squamous cells (image from IDEXX SediVue Dx™ Urine Sediment Analyzer).

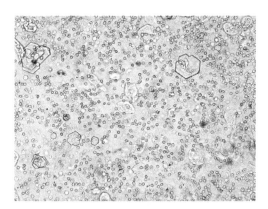

Figure 4.225 Cystine crystals, red blood cells, and squamous cells (image from IDEXX SediVue Dx™ Urine Sediment Analyzer).

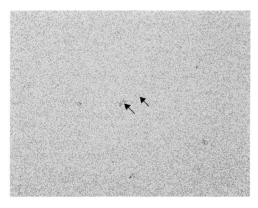

Figure 4.228 Cystine crystals (arrows) and hematuria in urine from a dog (100×).

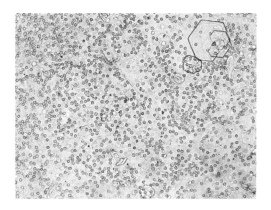

Figure 4.226 Cystine crystals and red blood cells (image from IDEXX SediVue Dx™ Urine Sediment Analyzer).

Figure 4.229 Cystine crystals and hematuria (100×).

Figure 4.230 Cystine crystals and hematuria (200×).

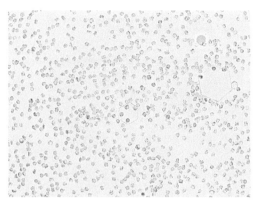

Figure 4.233 Cystine crystals and hematuria (500×).

Figure 4.231 Cystine crystals and hematuria (200×).

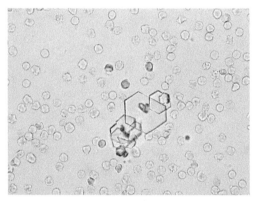

Figure 4.234 Cystine crystals and hematuria (1000×).

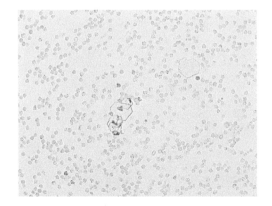

Figure 4.232 Cystine crystals and hematuria (500×).

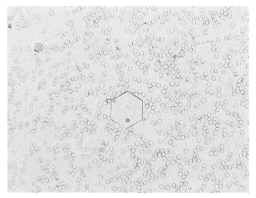

Figure 4.235 Cystine crystals and hematuria (500×).

Figure 4.236 Cystine crystals and hematuria (200×).

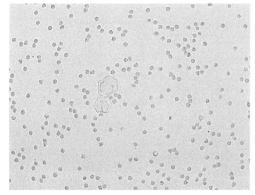

Figure 4.237 Cystine crystals and hematuria (500×).

Xanthine

Distinctive Features
Xanthine crystals are usually brown or yellow–brown. They may form variably sized spherules and cannot be reliably distinguished from some forms of ammonium urate and amorphous urate crystals by light microscopy. Infrared spectroscopy or high-pressure liquid chromatography can be used to identify xanthine crystals.

Diagnostic Significance
Xanthine crystalluria can occur secondary to allopurinol administration in dogs. Xanthine crystalluria has also been observed to occur as a result of a probable inborn error of purine metabolism in Cavalier King Charles spaniels and dachshunds. Naturally occurring xanthine crystalluria and xanthine uroliths have been observed in cats as a result of a suspected familial or congenital defect in xanthine oxidase activity (Osborne et al., 2004; Adams and Syme, 2010).

Next Steps
Investigate allopurinol administration, especially in dogs. If the patient has no history of allopurinol administration, investigate the potential for a hereditary or congenital condition. The potential for urolith formation should also be evaluated in patients with xanthine crystalluria. Increasing water con-

sumption in patients with xanthine crystalluria or urolith formation is recommended. In addition, a low-purine diet is recommended for patients receiving allopurinol for any reason, in order to reduce the potential for xanthine crystalluria development.

Amorphous (Phosphates, Urates, Xanthine, and Silicate)

Distinctive Features
These are small granular crystals without consistent distinctive features (Figures 4.238–4.248). They are present in many urine sediments. In alkaline urine, they are primarily phosphate crystals, while in acid urine, they are primarily urate crystals. Amorphous silicate and xanthine crystals can also occur. Amorphous crystals can be difficult to distinguish from degenerating cells and more distinct crystal formations that are also undergoing degeneration. In addition, amorphous crystals may be mistaken for bacterial cocci, but a Gram-stained or Romanowsky-type-stained preparation, such as Diff-Quik, should help in distinguishing bacteria from crystals.

Diagnostic Significance
Amorphous crystals are common and usually not diagnostically significant, although they may contribute to urolith formation in dogs and cats. Radiodense silicate uroliths, which

classically take on a jackstone appearance, may occasionally form from silicate crystals, especially in the German shepherd dog.

Next Steps

If patient history or clinical findings give any suggestion of urolith formation, additional procedures may be indicated, such as diagnostic imaging. If uncertain about the presence of amorphous crystals versus bacterial cocci, a urine sediment sample that has been Gram-stained or stained with a Romanowsky-type stain, such as Diff-Quik, should be examined. Increasing patient water consumption could be considered.

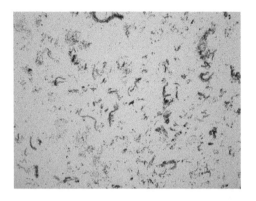

Figure 4.238 Amorphous crystals (urate, phosphates, and silicates) are small and without consistent distinctive features (100×).

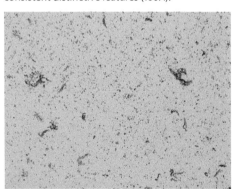

Figure 4.239 Amorphous crystals (100×).

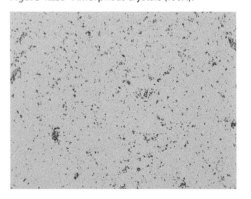

Figure 4.240 Amorphous crystals (100×).

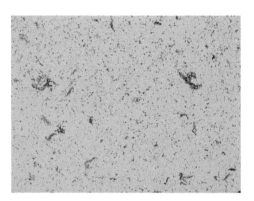

Figure 4.241 Amorphous crystals (100×).

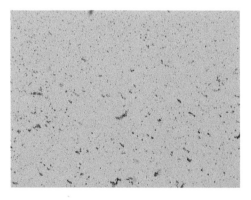

Figure 4.242 Amorphous crystals (100×).

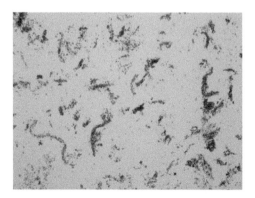

Figure 4.243 Amorphous crystals (200×).

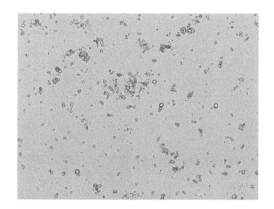

Figure 4.244   Amorphous crystals (200×).

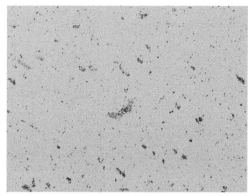

Figure 4.247   Amorphous crystals (200×).

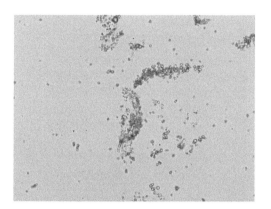

Figure 4.245   Amorphous crystals (500×).

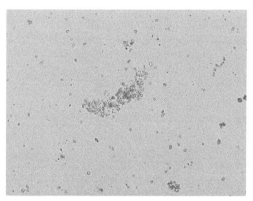

Figure 4.248   Amorphous crystals (500×).

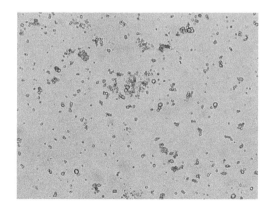

Figure 4.246   Amorphous crystals (500×).

Crystals Not Typically Associated with Canine and Feline Urolith Formation

Tyrosine and Leucine

Distinctive Features

Tyrosine crystals occur as refractile needles. The needles may be present individually, in clusters, or in sheaves. Leucine crystals are yellowish brown, round structures with radial striations.

Diagnostic Significance

Tyrosine and leucine crystals are only very rarely seen in dogs and cats. Severe hepatoinsufficiency in which amino acid metabolism is impaired has been associated with tyrosine and leucine crystal formation in humans. Tyrosine crystals have occasionally accompanied leucine crystals in human patients with hepatic disorders. To the authors' knowledge no reports of feline or canine tyrosine or leucine uroliths in the United States have been published. At least one major urolith center (University of Minnesota) in the United States has never identified a tyrosine or leucine urolith. It may be more accurate to refer to feline or canine crystals with the characteristics of tyrosine or leucine as tyrosine- or leucine-like crystals since the actual presence of tyrosine or leucine compounds in such crystals has never been verified (Personal communication with Dr. Jody Lulich, University of Minnesota, June, 2016).

Next Steps

Patient history, clinical signs, clinical chemistry, and hematology results should be reviewed for evidence of hepatic disease. If the appearance of tyrosine- or leucine-like crystals is persistent or unexplained, urinary tract signs of illness are present, consultation with a veterinary clinical pathologist or urology expert may be advisable.

Bilirubin

Distinctive Features

Bilirubin crystals (Figures 4.249–4.283) are golden to golden-brown, needle-like crystals that often form clusters resembling pine needles. Bilirubin crystals with adhered lipid droplets at the distal tip are sometimes referred to as flashlight bilirubin crystals (Figure 4.284).

Diagnostic Significance

Bilirubin crystals are composed of conjugated bilirubin which is freely filterable through the renal glomeruli. An occasional bilirubin crystal may be observed in urine sediment from normal dogs with highly concentrated urine.

Moderate to abundant numbers of bilirubin crystals suggest hepatic or post-hepatic biliary disease. If biliary disease is the cause of the bilirubin crystalluria, plasma/serum bilirubin concentration will be increased.

Next Steps

Patient history, clinical signs, clinical chemistry, and hematology results should be reviewed for evidence of hepatobiliary disease.

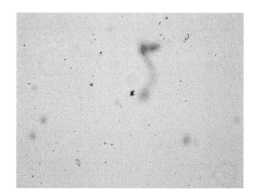

Figure 4.249 Urine from a dog. Aggregate of bilirubin crystals (100×).

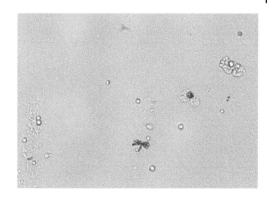

Figure 4.252 Aggregate of bilirubin crystals (200×).

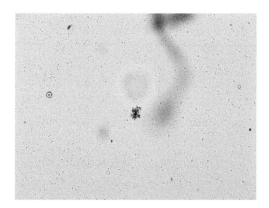

Figure 4.250 Aggregate of bilirubin crystals (200×).

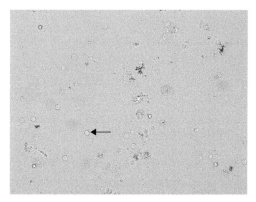

Figure 4.253 Aggregate of bilirubin crystals and white blood cells (arrow) (100×).

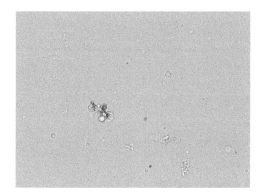

Figure 4.251 Urine from a cat. Aggregate of bilirubin crystals (200×).

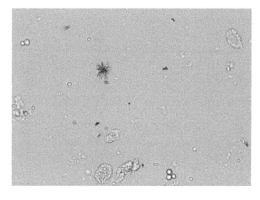

Figure 4.254 Aggregate of bilirubin crystals (200×).

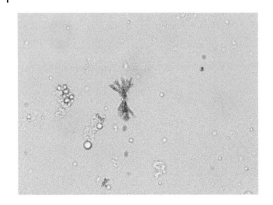

Figure 4.255 Aggregate of bilirubin crystals (600×).

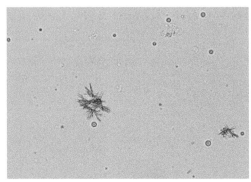

Figure 4.258 Aggregate of bilirubin crystals (600×).

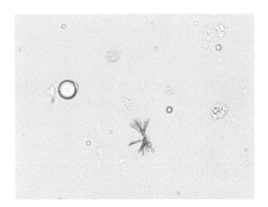

Figure 4.256 Aggregate of bilirubin crystals (600×).

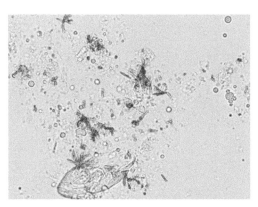

Figure 4.259 Several aggregates of bilirubin crystals (200×).

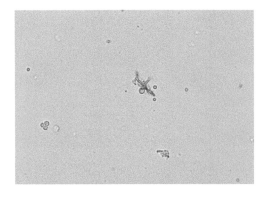

Figure 4.257 Aggregate of bilirubin crystals (600×).

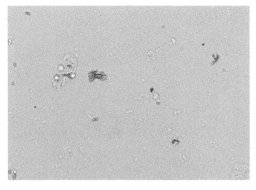

Figure 4.260 Aggregate of bilirubin crystals (200×).

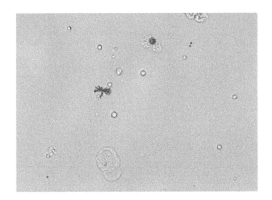

Figure 4.261 Aggregate of bilirubin crystals (100×).

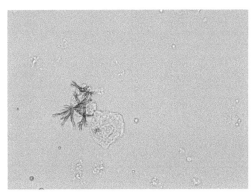

Figure 4.264 Aggregate of bilirubin crystals overlying squamous cells (600×).

Figure 4.262 Aggregates of bilirubin crystals (100×).

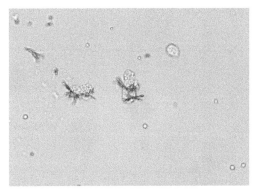

Figure 4.265 Aggregates of bilirubin crystals (600×).

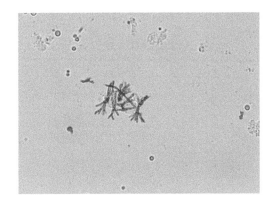

Figure 4.263 Aggregate of bilirubin crystals (600×).

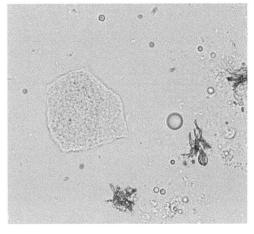

Figure 4.266 Aggregates of bilirubin crystals, bilirubin-stained squamous cell (600×).

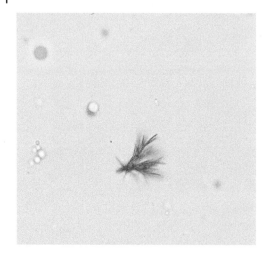

Figure 4.267 Aggregate of bilirubin crystals (600×).

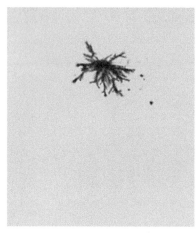

Figure 4.270 Aggregate of bilirubin crystals (1000×).

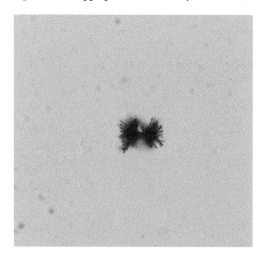

Figure 4.268 Aggregate of bilirubin crystals (600×).

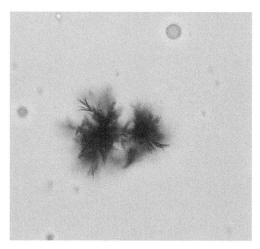

Figure 4.271 Aggregate of bilirubin crystals (1000×).

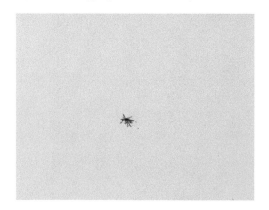

Figure 4.269 Urine from a cat. Aggregate of bilirubin crystals (100×).

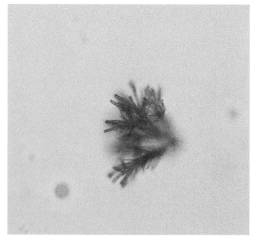

Figure 4.272 Aggregate of bilirubin crystals (1000×).

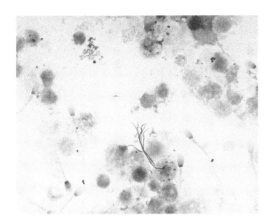

Figure 4.273 Urine from a dog. Aggregate of bilirubin crystals, deteriorating RBCs and sperm (Wright stain; 500×).

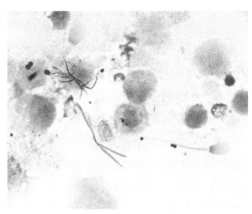

Figure 4.276 Aggregate of bilirubin crystals (Wright stain; 1000×).

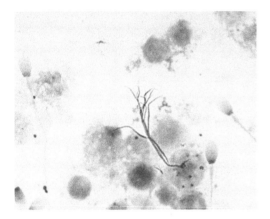

Figure 4.274 Aggregate of bilirubin crystals (Wright stain; 1000×).

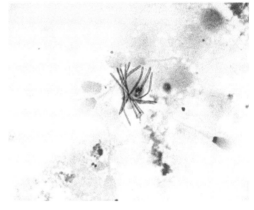

Figure 4.277 Aggregate of bilirubin crystals (Wright stain; 1000×).

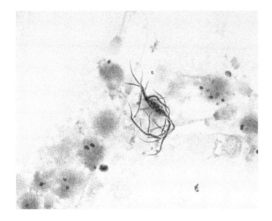

Figure 4.275 Aggregate of bilirubin crystals (Wright stain; 1000×).

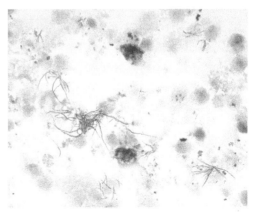

Figure 4.278 Aggregate of bilirubin crystals (Wright stain; 1000×).

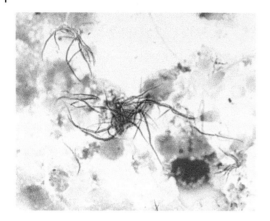

Figure 4.279 Aggregate of bilirubin crystals (Wright stain; 1000×).

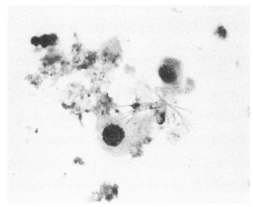

Figure 4.282 Aggregate of bilirubin crystals and deteriorating cells (Wright stain; 500×).

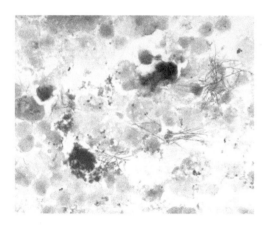

Figure 4.280 Aggregate of bilirubin crystals (Wright stain; 1000×).

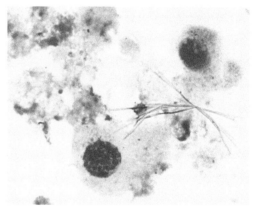

Figure 4.283 Aggregate of bilirubin crystals (Wright stain; 1000×).

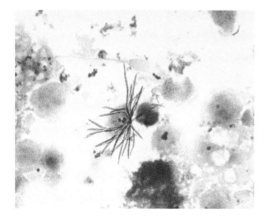

Figure 4.281 Aggregate of bilirubin crystals (Wright stain; 1000×).

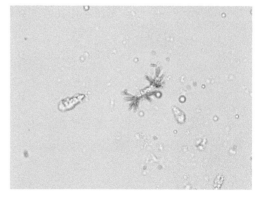

Figure 4.284 Urine from a cat. Aggregate of bilirubin crystals with adhered lipid droplet giving it a "flashlight" appearance (600×).

Melamine/Melamine Cyanurate

Distinctive Features
Melamine/melamine cyanurate crystals are brown to yellow–brown, small, and round, with radiating striations from the center (Figures 4.285–4.291).

Diagnostic Significance
Melamine crystals, when precipitated in combination with cyanuric acid, may indicate potential toxicity and acute renal failure as in past occurrences where pet food contaminated with melamine/cyanuric acid has been ingested.

Next Steps
In addition to performing a complete urinalysis, patient history (including food history), clinical signs, clinical chemistry, and hematology results should be reviewed for evidence of acute kidney disease and potential toxin exposure.

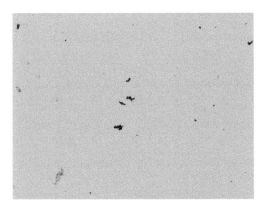

Figure 4.285 Urine from a cat. Aggregates of melamine crystals (100×). Melamine/melamine cyanurate crystals are small, round, yellow to brown.

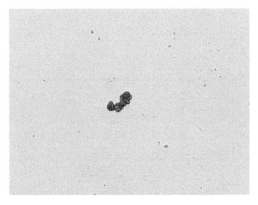

Figure 4.287 Aggregates of melamine crystals (500×). Internal radiating striations are visible with higher magnification.

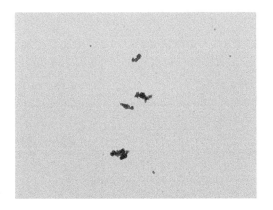

Figure 4.286 Aggregates of melamine crystals (200×).

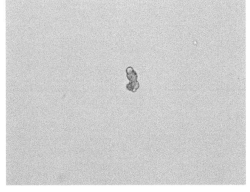

Figure 4.288 Aggregates of melamine crystals (1000×).

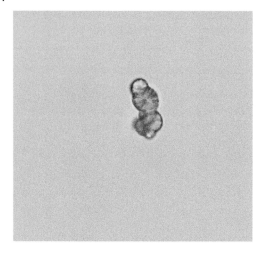

Figure 4.289 Aggregates of melamine crystals (1000×).

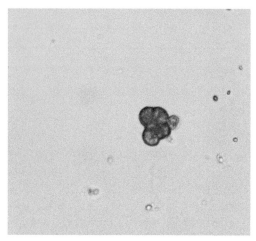

Figure 4.291 Aggregate of melamine crystals (1000×).

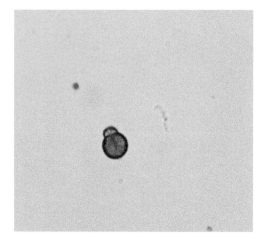

Figure 4.290 Melamine crystals (1000×).

Cholesterol

Distinctive Features
Cholesterol crystals appear as large, clear, rectangular, flat plates, often with a notch in the corner (Figure 4.292–4.296).

Diagnostic Significance
Cholesterol crystals are rarely observed in animals and therefore their significance is undetermined. Although cholesterol crystals may be observed in clinically normal dogs, there can be a possible association with excessive cellular degeneration or with protein-losing nephropathy (PLN). Urinalysis findings in patients with PLN may also include a positive urine chemistry result for protein and microscopic findings of casts (usually hyaline but may be granular, waxy or fatty), fat droplets, and misshapen erythrocytes (due to passage through damaged glomerular capillaries).

Next Steps
Patient history, clinical signs, and clinical chemistry results should be reviewed for evidence of PLN.

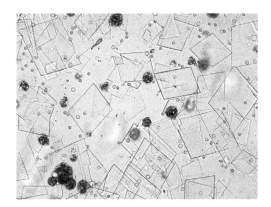

Figure 4.292 Cholesterol crystals appear as large, clear, flat plates often with a notch in the corner. Red blood cells are in the background (image from IDEXX SediVue Dx™ Urine Sediment Analyzer).

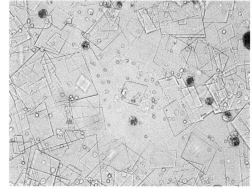

Figure 4.295 Cholesterol crystals (image from IDEXX SediVue Dx™ Urine Sediment Analyzer).

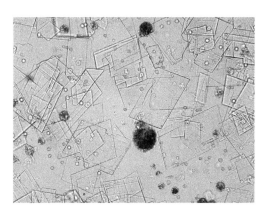

Figure 4.293 Cholesterol crystals (image from IDEXX SediVue Dx™ Urine Sediment Analyzer).

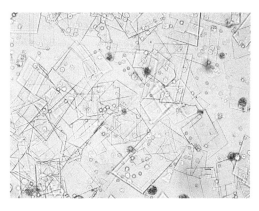

Figure 4.296 Cholesterol crystals (image from IDEXX SediVue Dx™ Urine Sediment Analyzer).

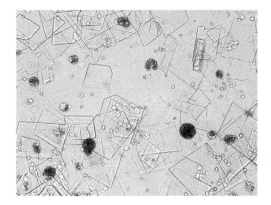

Figure 4.294 Cholesterol crystals (image from IDEXX SediVue Dx™ Urine Sediment Analyzer).

Drug-Induced Crystals

Observation of unknown urine crystals should prompt review of the patient's history, including known drug administration or potential exposure to drugs.

Sulfonamides

Distinctive Features
A variety of crystals may occur due to therapeutic administration of sulfonamides. They generally occur as fuzzy, brown needle-like crystals in sheaves or rosettes. They may also occur as globules with radial striations, wedge-shaped structures with one sharp point and pronounced serrated (saw tooth) edges on one or both sides, and transparent oval crystals with serrations on one or both edges (Figures 4.297–4.299).

Diagnostic Significance
Sulfonamide crystalluria indicates that sulfonamides have been administered. The cur-

rent sulfa drugs are highly soluble and urinary sulfa crystal formation is usually associated with sulfonamide overdose.

Next Steps
If there is a question as to whether or not the crystals are actually sulfonamide crystals, the lignin test may be done. In this test, one to two drops of urine sediment is put on a piece of newspaper (crude cellulose) and a drop of 10% hydrochloric acid is put on top of the drop of urine sediment. If sulfonamide crystals are present, a yellow to orange color forms immediately. As a control, a drop of 10% hydrochloric acid is placed on the newspaper without urine. If sulfonamide crystals are present in the urine and a sulfa drug is currently being administered to the patient, the dosage regimen should be reviewed.

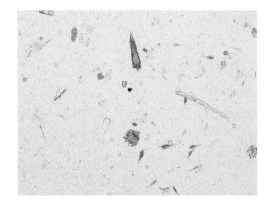

Figure 4.297 Sulfa crystals (200×).

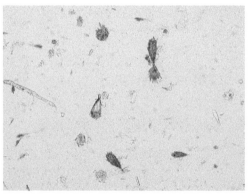

Figure 4.298 Sulfa crystals (200×).

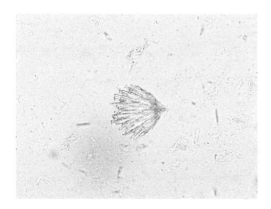

Figure 4.299 Sulfa crystals (500×).

Ampicillin

Distinctive Features
Ampicillin crystals occur as long, thin needles or prisms. Osborne and Stevens (1999) reported observing wheat sheaf-like crystals in the urine of a dog that had been given large doses of ampicillin.

Diagnostic Significance
No significance other than association with ampicillin administration.

Next Steps
None required.

Radiopaque Contrast Agents

Distinctive Features
Long, colorless, pointed, needle-like crystals have been observed in canine urine (Osborne and Stevens, 1999) containing sodium diatrizoate (Hypaque 50) and flat rectangular plates have been seen in urine containing diatrizoate meglumine (Renografin). Sodium diatrizoate crystals can be differentiated from sulfa crystals by the lignin test described previously under "Sulfonamides".

Diagnostic Significance
No significance other than association with administration of radiopaque contrast agent.

Next Steps
None required.

Cells

Many different cell types (superficial squamous cells, transitional cells, caudate epithelial cells, renal tubular cells, leukocytes, erythrocytes, and neoplastic cells) can be seen in urine sediment. The morphology, frequency, and significance of each of these cell types are briefly discussed here.

Transitional Epithelial Cells

Distinctive Features
While transitional epithelial cells (Figures 4.300–4.321) vary tremendously in size and shape, they are generally medium-sized, round, oval, to polygonal cells with a large round to oval nucleus that is often centrally located. Their cytoplasm appears granular. They may be present individually or in groups. Occasional binucleated cells may be observed. Transitional cells are typically two to four times larger than WBCs although distinction between WBCs and small transitional cells is nearly impossible on unstained preparations. An air-dried smear of urine sediment stained with one of the rapid stains (e.g. Diff-Quik) would be needed to characterize the population of cells if there is doubt.

Diagnostic Significance
Transitional epithelial cells are the normal lining cells of the urinary tract from the renal pelvis to the proximal urethra. They

are a normal finding in urine sediment, and noncatheterized urine samples from normal dogs and cats generally contain a low number of transitional epithelial cells. Causes of high numbers of transitional epithelial cells include catheterized urine samples, cystoliths, inflammation (infectious or noninfectious), neoplasia, and chemical irritation (some chemotherapy agents).

Caudate epithelial cells are a type of transitional epithelial cell that line the renal pelvis. They may have a somewhat triangular, tapered, tail-like, or caudate shape and may be difficult to differentiate from distorted transitional epithelial cells, especially in catheterized samples. The presence of renal caudate epithelial cells indicates increased sloughing of renal pelvic cells as occurs with pyelonephritis. However, recognizing epithelial cells as caudate epithelial cells is difficult and is generally considered unreliable unless the examiner is very experienced.

Next Steps
If the epithelial cells appear abnormal or are increased in number, an air-dried slide of urine sediment should be sent to a clinical pathologist/cytologist for evaluation. Investigation of the patient's history, clinical signs, clinical chemistry, hematology, and urinalysis, with or without renal ultrasonography, and urine culture should be carried out for evidence of pyelonephritis.

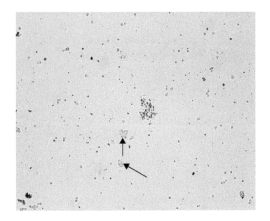

Figure 4.300 Urine sediment from a cat. A few small aggregates of transitional cells (arrows) (100×).

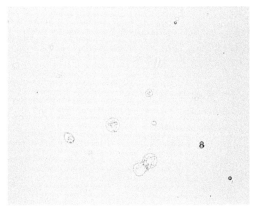

Figure 4.302 Urine sediment from a cat. Transitional cells (500×).

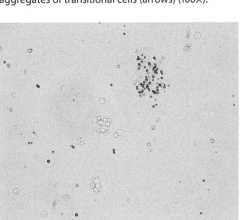

Figure 4.301 Small aggregates of transitional cells (200×).

Figure 4.303 Small group of transitional cells (100×).

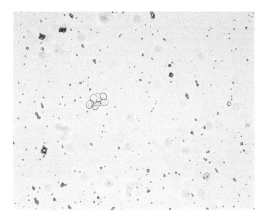

Figure 4.304 Transitional cells (200×).

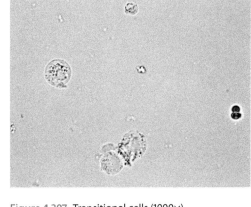

Figure 4.307 Transitional cells (1000×).

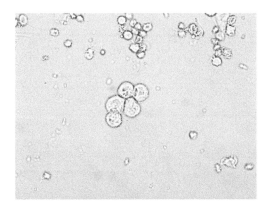

Figure 4.305 Transitional cells (1000×).

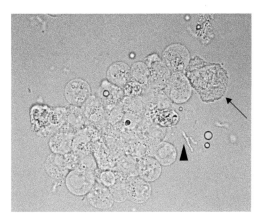

Figure 4.308 Urine sediment from a cat. Aggregate of transitional cells, squamous cell (arrow), and bacteria (arrow head) (1000×).

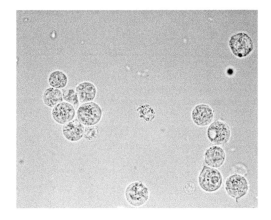

Figure 4.306 Transitional cells (1000×).

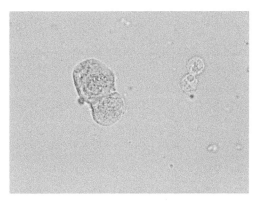

Figure 4.309 Transitional cells and two WBCs. Transitional cells are typically larger than WBCs (1000×).

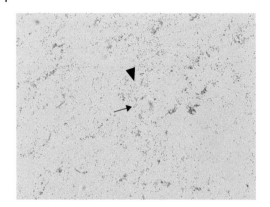

Figure 4.310 Transitional cells (arrow), squamous cells (arrow head), and RBCs. There are many cells in this urine sediment, but at this magnification it is difficult to distinguish what they are (100×).

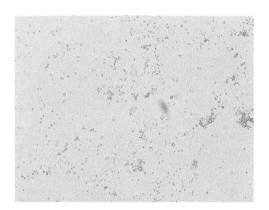

Figure 4.311 Transitional cells, squamous cells, and RBCs (200×).

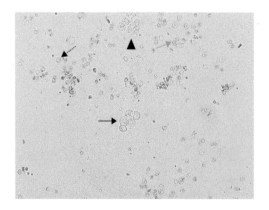

Figure 4.312 Transitional cells (black arrow), squamous cells (arrow head), WBCs (dotted arrow), RBCs (blue arrow) (500×).

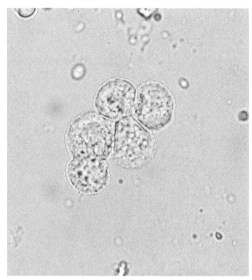

Figure 4.313 Transitional cells (1000×).

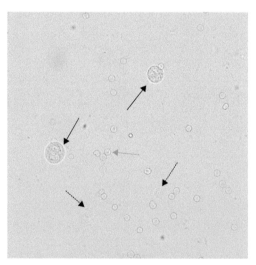

Figure 4.314 Transitional cells (arrows), WBC (dotted arrows), RBCs (blue arrow) (500×).

Figure 4.315 Transitional cell and debris (supravital urine stain; 500×).

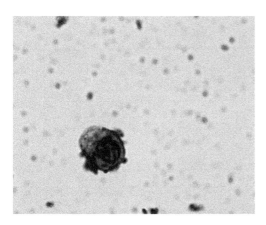

Figure 4.316 Transitional cell (supravital urine stain; 1000×).

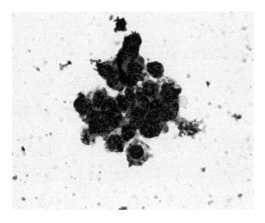

Figure 4.317 An aggregate of transitional cells (supravital urine stain;1000×).

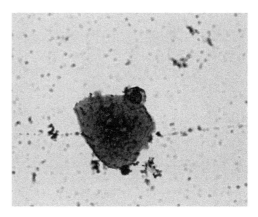

Figure 4.318 Transitional cell and squamous cell (supravital urine stain; 1000×).

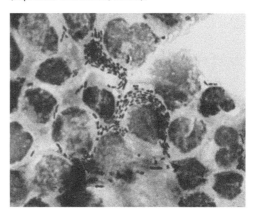

Figure 4.319 Urine sample from a cat. These cells are deteriorated and no longer identifiable. There are moderate numbers of bacterial rods (Wright stain; 1000×).

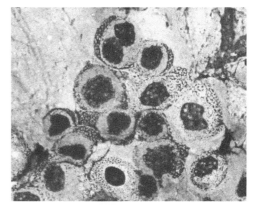

Figure 4.320 Urine sample from a dog. The transitional cells are deteriorating; their nuclear chromatin is lacey, and their cytoplasm is stippled. Most cells deteriorate quickly in urine (Wright stain; 1000×).

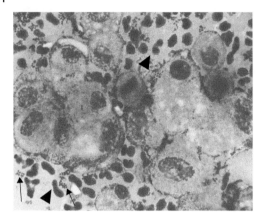

Figure 4.321 Deteriorating transitional cells and other cells, possibly leukocytes (arrow heads), bacterial cocci (arrows) (Wright stain; 1000×).

Squamous Epithelial Cells

Distinctive Features

Urine samples may contain nonkeratinized and/or keratinized squamous epithelial cells (Figures 4.322–4.342). Nonkeratinized squamous cells originate in the distal urethra, prepuce, or vagina. They can vary in size from medium-sized, round cells to larger flat cells with polygonal cytoplasm, and typically have a small round nucleus. The medium-sized nonkeratinized cells can be difficult to distinguish from larger transitional cells. An air-dried, stained preparation is often needed to characterize these cells further. Keratinized squamous cells originate from external skin. These are large, flat cells with an abundant amount of angular cytoplasm and, if the nucleus is present, it is small and round. They are often seen individually but can occur in sheets. Occasionally, "rolled-up" cells, called keratin bars, may be observed. These cells are cylindrical and should not be confused with casts.

Diagnostic Significance

Superficial squamous epithelial cells typically occur in urine sediment due to contamination from the urethra, vagina, or skin, and are most commonly seen in catheterized and voided urine samples. Superficial squamous epithelial cells are an incidental finding and are usually of no diagnostic significance.

Large numbers of squamous cells can occasionally be associated with squamous metaplasia of the canine prostate, resulting from either an exogenous estrogen source or an estrogen-secreting testicular tumor.

Next Steps

If a large number of squamous cells is observed in the urine of a male dog, review the history, physical findings, and hematologic laboratory work to determine if any evidence of testicular tumor or exogenous estrogen exposure exists.

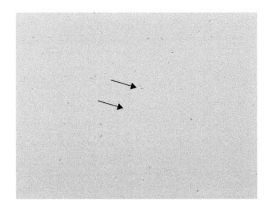

Figure 4.322 This urine sediment is poorly cellular with a few squamous cells (arrows) (100×).

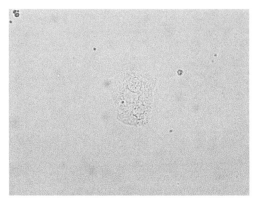

Figure 4.325 Squamous cell (1000×).

Figure 4.323 At higher magnification squamous cells are readily identified (200×).

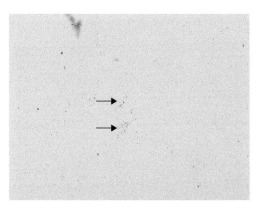

Figure 4.326 Squamous cells (arrows) (100×).

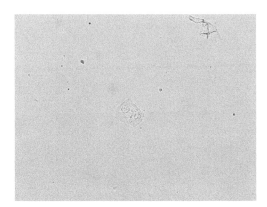

Figure 4.324 Squamous cells. The cell in the upper right corner is folded (500×).

Figure 4.327 Squamous cells (200×).

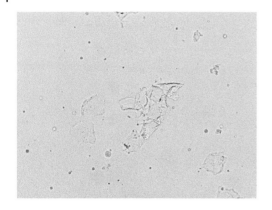

Figure 4.328 An aggregate of squamous cells in the center and individual polygonal squamous cells (500×).

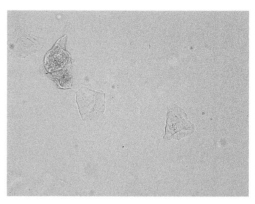

Figure 4.331 Squamous cells (image from IDEXX SediVue Dx™ Urine Sediment Analyzer).

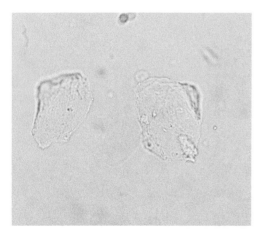

Figure 4.329 Squamous cells (1000×).

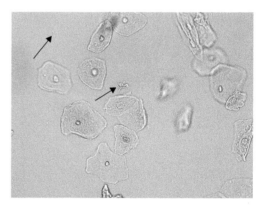

Figure 4.332 Squamous cells and background contaminant bacterial rods (arrow) (image from IDEXX SediVue Dx™ Urine Sediment Analyzer).

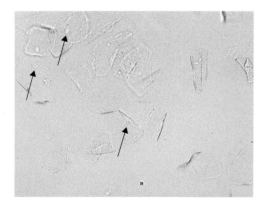

Figure 4.330 Squamous cells. Some have a small visible nucleus (arrows) (image from IDEXX SediVue Dx™ Urine Sediment Analyzer).

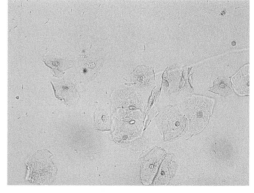

Figure 4.333 Squamous cells and background bacteria (image from IDEXX SediVue Dx™ Urine Sediment Analyzer).

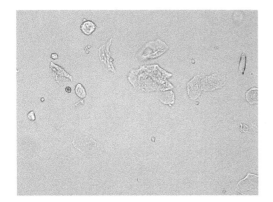

Figure 4.334 Squamous cells (image from IDEXX SediVue Dx™ Urine Sediment Analyzer).

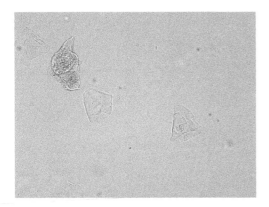

Figure 4.335 Squamous cells (image from IDEXX SediVue Dx™ Urine Sediment Analyzer).

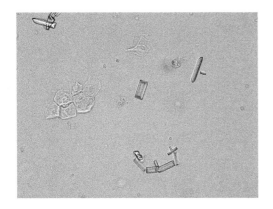

Figure 4.336 Squamous cells and struvite crystals (image from IDEXX SediVue Dx™ Urine Sediment Analyzer).

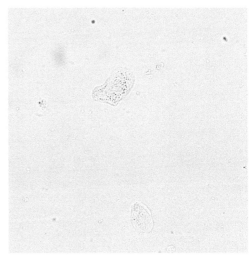

Figure 4.337 Squamous cells and background bacteria (1000×).

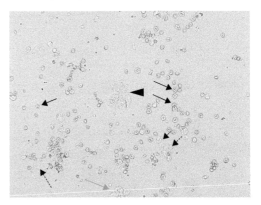

Figure 4.338 Aggregate of squamous cells (arrow head), RBCs (arrows), WBCs (dotted arrows), and transitional cells (blue arrow) (500×).

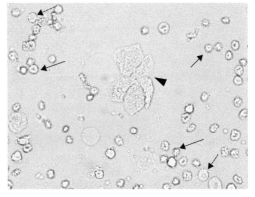

Figure 4.339 Aggregate of squamous cells (arrow head), RBCs (arrows), WBC, and bacteria (dotted arrows) (1000×).

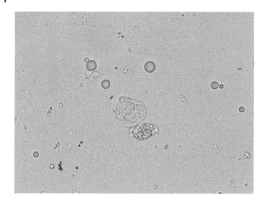

Figure 4.340 Urine from an icteric cat. Bilirubin-stained squamous cells and lipid droplets (600×).

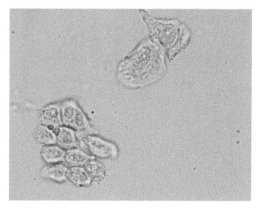

Figure 4.342 Squamous cells (upper right) and cluster of transitional cells (1000×).

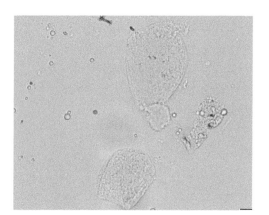

Figure 4.341 Bilirubin-stained squamous cells and lipid droplets (1000×).

Renal Tubular (Cuboidal) Epithelial Cells

Distinctive Features

Renal tubular cells are small cells (slightly larger than a neutrophil) that are typically round with a round to oval, eccentrically placed nucleus. Renal tubular cells from cats and diabetic dogs frequently contain many small to a few large fat globules. Renal epithelial cells that do not contain fat may be difficult or impossible to differentiate from small transitional epithelial cells. Differentiation of renal epithelial cells from leukocytes is based on their size and nuclear shape and is enhanced by staining the urine sediment so that the nuclear shape can be better distinguished.

Diagnostic Significance

Renal tubular cells may be found in urine sediment from normal animals. Moderate to high numbers of renal tubular epithelial cells suggest acute renal tubular injury.

Next Steps

If moderate to high numbers of renal tubular cells are observed, review the patient's history, physical exam findings, CBC, biochemistry profile, and urinalysis results for evidence of acute renal disease.

Leukocytes

Distinctive Features

Neutrophils comprise the vast majority of leukocytes seen in urine sediment. Leukocytes are spherical and colorless with grainy-appearing cytoplasm; occasionally the lobulated shape of the nucleus can be discerned (Figures 4.343–4.365). Leukocytes may aggregate but are generally present as individual cells. They are larger than erythrocytes (one-and-a-half to two times larger) and usually smaller than transitional cells. The distinction between transitional epithelial cells and WBCs may be ambiguous, particularly if there is delay in examining the urine as WBCs can swell and appear larger. An air-dried, stained preparation should be examined if there is doubt.

While leukocyte type cannot be readily distinguished in unstained urine sediment specimens, they are presumed to be neutrophils, although low numbers of small lymphocytes and macrophages are sometimes present. An air-dried, stained preparation would be needed to cytologically characterize individual leukocytes.

Leukocytes shrink in hypertonic urine and swell or, sometimes, lyse in hypotonic urine or very alkaline urine. Leukocytes in urine are also referred to as "glitter" cells because their intracytoplasmic granules refract light creating a "glitter" or refractile appearance to the cell. This is especially pronounced in hypotonic urine, because the leukocyte swells and its granules undergo Brownian motion. Crenated erythrocytes may also "glitter." However, the "glitter" of erythrocytes can be recognized as arising from the external surface of the cell (the echinocyte projections), whereas, the "glitter" from leukocytes can be recognized as arising from inside the cell.

Diagnostic Significance

A few WBCs may be present in the urine of healthy dogs and cats. While the number of acceptable WBCs in urine sediment varies with the collection technique (voided, catheterized, or cystocentesis samples), generally 5 WBC/hpf is considered the upper limit of the reference range for healthy animals. Increased numbers of neutrophils (pyuria) indicate inflammation of the urinary tract or contamination from the genital tract. The inflammation may be of infectious or noninfectious origin. White cell aggregation may be seen with chronic inflammation and occurs more often with bacterial infections.

Next Steps

A careful search for bacteria should be performed: however, bacteria are not always found microscopically, even when a bacterial infection is the cause of the inflammation. Additional recommendations include: investigation of the urinary system for the site of inflammation; review of hematology and chemistry profiles for evidence of systemic inflammatory effect; culture and sensitivity of urine to aid in diagnosis and guide therapy.

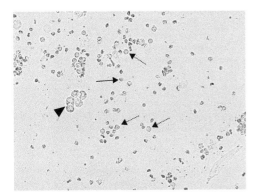

Figure 4.343 Urine from a dog with RBCs (arrow), WBCs (dotted arrows), and transitional cells (arrow head) (200×).

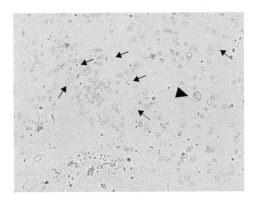

Figure 4.344 An active urine sediment from a dog with numerous crenated RBCs (blue arrows), WBCs (black arrows), a single transitional cell (arrow head) and bacteria (dotted arrows) (200×).

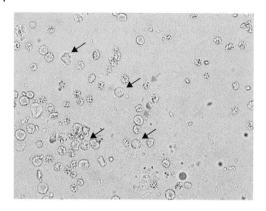

Figure 4.345 White blood cells (black arrows) are slightly larger than RBCs (blue arrows) and often have a grainy appearance (600×).

Figure 4.348 Numerous WBCs and bacteria (image from IDEXX SediVue Dx™ Urine Sediment Analyzer).

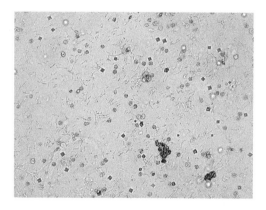

Figure 4.346 WBCs, bacteria, and calcium oxalate dihydrate crystals (image from IDEXX SediVue Dx™ Urine Sediment Analyzer).

Figure 4.349 WBCs and bacteria (image from IDEXX SediVue Dx™ Urine Sediment Analyzer).

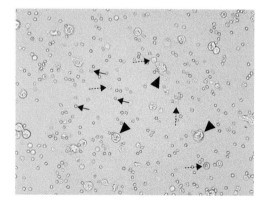

Figure 4.347 RBCs (arrows), WBCs (dotted arrows), and transitional cells (arrow head) (image from IDEXX SediVue Dx™ Urine Sediment Analyzer).

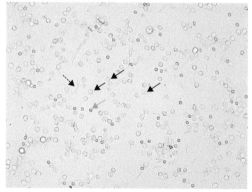

Figure 4.350 Numerous WBCs (black arrows), RBCs (blue arrow), and bacteria (dashed arrow) (image from IDEXX SediVue Dx™ Urine Sediment Analyzer).

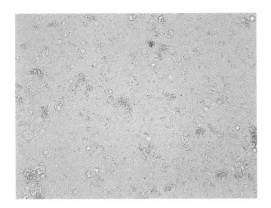

Figure 4.351 WBCs and bacteria (image from IDEXX SediVue Dx™ Urine Sediment Analyzer).

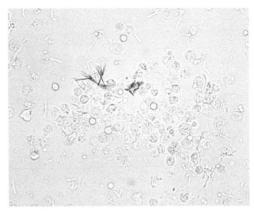

Figure 4.354 WBCs, a few transitional cells, bacteria, and bilirubin crystals (1000×).

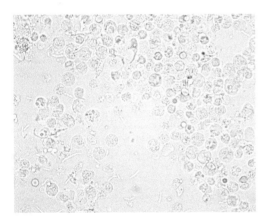

Figure 4.352 Numerous WBCs and bacteria (1000×).

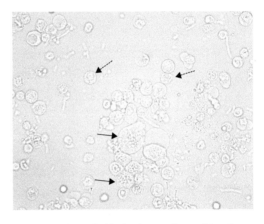

Figure 4.355 WBCs (dashed arrows), transitional cells (arrows), and bacteria (1000×).

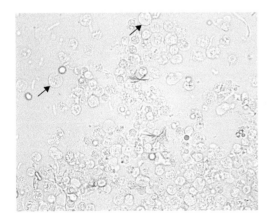

Figure 4.353 Numerous WBCs, a few transitional cells (arrows), bacteria, and bilirubin crystals (1000×).

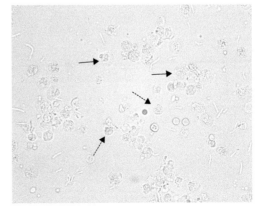

Figure 4.356 WBCs (dashed arrows), transitional cells (arrows), and bacteria. WBCs are usually smaller than transitional cells (1000×).

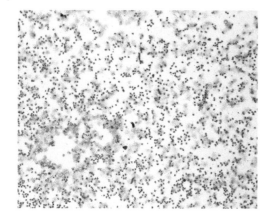

Figure 4.357 Urine from a cat. Deteriorating leukocytes (Wright stain; 100×).

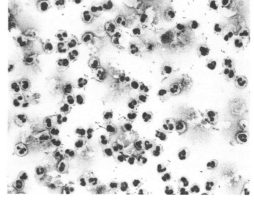

Figure 4.360 Degenerate neutrophils and bacteria (Wright stain; 500×).

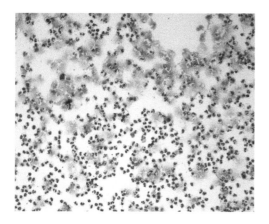

Figure 4.358 Numerous degenerate neutrophils (Wright stain; 200×).

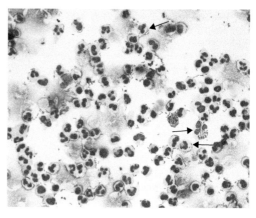

Figure 4.361 Degenerate neutrophils, some with intracellular bacteria (arrows), and numerous background bacteria (Wright stain; 500×).

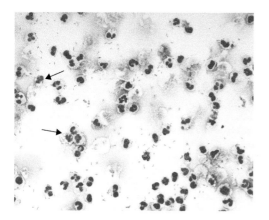

Figure 4.359 Degenerate neutrophils, some with intracellular bacteria (arrows), and numerous background bacteria (Wright stain; 500×).

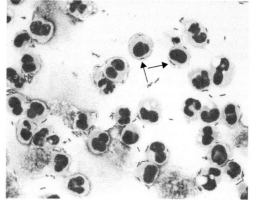

Figure 4.362 Degenerate neutrophils, some with intracellular bacteria (arrows), and numerous background bacteria (Wright stain; 1000×).

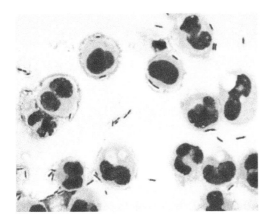

Figure 4.363 Degenerate neutrophils with intracellular bacteria (Wright stain; 1000×).

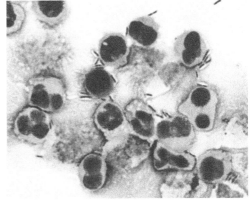

Figure 4.365 Degenerate neutrophils with intracellular bacteria (Wright stain; 1000×).

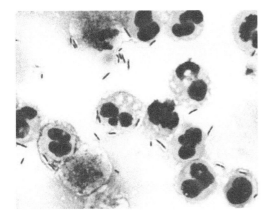

Figure 4.364 Degenerate neutrophils with intracellular bacteria (Wright stain; 1000×).

Erythrocytes

Distinctive Features

Depending on the osmolality of the urine, erythrocyte morphology will vary from crenated to normal to swollen to ruptured (Figures 4.366–4.374). In general, erythrocytes are small, pale, round, biconcave discs that have no nucleus.

In concentrated urine the erythrocytes will be smaller and often appear crenated due to RBC water loss into the hypertonic urine environment. Crenated erythrocytes appear pale and spherical with irregular surface projections. Crenated erythrocytes may "glitter" due to light refraction from the projec-

tions. They can be distinguished from leukocytes because leukocytes are larger. The "glitter" from leukocytes is from within the cell instead of from the surface.

In isotonic urine the erythrocytes often have a normal RBC morphology. Therefore, they appear pale and round, with a smooth border and often a biconcave appearance.

In hypotonic urine erythrocytes swell and may lyse. Swollen erythrocytes appear like normal erythrocytes only larger and not biconcave. Lysed erythrocytes may appear as faint, colorless circles (ghost cells) or may become transparent and not be visible.

It is important not to misidentify lipid droplets as RBCs in unstained urine. Lipid droplets can be differentiated from RBCs because lipid droplets vary markedly in size and float, causing them to be in a different plane of focus (just below the coverslip). Using fine focusing, the biconcave shape of the RBC is apparent.

Diagnostic Significance

A few RBCs may be present in urine of healthy dogs and cats. While the number of acceptable RBCs in urine sediment varies with the collection technique (voided, manual compression, catheterized, or cystocentesis samples), generally 5 RBC/hpf is considered the upper limit of reference range for healthy animals.

Hematuria (an increased number of erythrocytes in urine) indicates hemorrhage into the urinary system. If the urine was collected by free catch, the hemorrhage may be anywhere in the urogenital system. However, when RBCs appear primarily in the latter part of urination from urine collected by free catch (see Chapter 1, section on "Free-Catch Urine Collection"), the bladder is often the source of hematuria. Hematuria in urine collected by urinary bladder catheterization or cystocentesis suggests that hemorrhage is occurring from the urinary bladder, ureters, renal pelvis, or kidney.

It should be kept in mind that hematuria, particularly microscopic hematuria, can be caused by the urine collection technique itself, especially when catheterization or cystocentesis has been used in obtaining the specimen.

Next Steps

Review the patient's history and physical examination findings to further characterize micturition and associated hematuria, as well as to establish whether any evidence of coagulopathy exists. Additional investigation of the urinary system, including diagnostic imaging, may be indicated to determine the site of hemorrhage. The hematology profile should be examined to determine extent of hemorrhage (i.e. whether the hematocrit is low), identify any evidence of systemic inflammation, and evaluate platelet numbers. The reader is referred to an algorithmic reference for more complete guidelines of the diagnosis of hematuria (Bowles, 2008).

Figure 4.366 Numerous RBCs (100×).

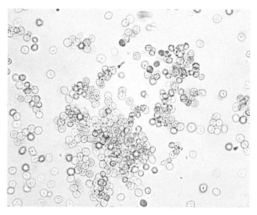

Figure 4.367 RBCs are biconcave and often appear with an internal ring or "donut shaped" in urine sediment (200×).

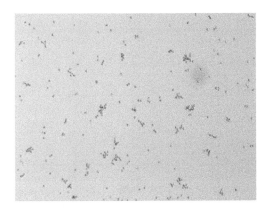

Figure 4.368 Numerous RBCs (100×).

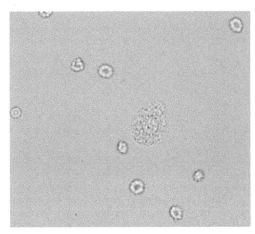

Figure 4.371 RBCs and squamous cell (600×).

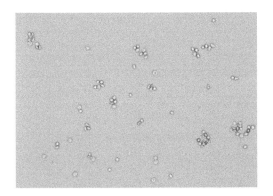

Figure 4.369 RBCs (200×).

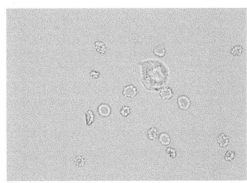

Figure 4.372 RBCs and squamous cell (600×).

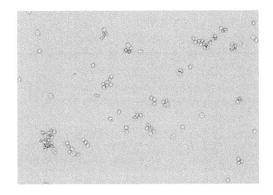

Figure 4.370 RBCs (200×).

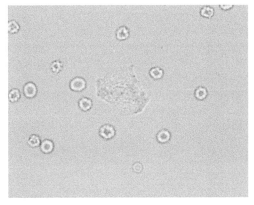

Figure 4.373 RBCs and squamous cell (600×).

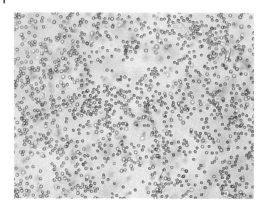

Figure 4.374 Numerous RBCs and a few squamous cells (image from IDEXX SediVue Dx™ Urine Sediment Analyzer).

Atypical (Neoplastic) Cells

Distinctive Features

Atypical cells are occasionally observed in urine sediment, especially those of transitional epithelial origin (Figures 4.375–4.384, 4.392–4.400, 4.412–4.418). However, most urine samples from animals with bladder tumors do not contain sufficient numbers of atypical cells for a cytologic diagnosis. When sufficient numbers are present and atypical cells are observed, it is best to make an air-dried smear of the urine sediment and stain it with any of the Romanowsky-type stains such as Diff-Quik (Figures 4.385–4.391, 4.401–4.411, 4.419–4.421). Normal transitional cells may contain small, smooth, round nucleoli. However, if marked cellular atypia (especially in the absence of inflammation) is present, neoplasia should be suspected.

Diagnostic Significance

Identification of unusual cells in urine may indicate a neoplasm within the urinary system. Often the type of neoplasm can be identified by an experienced cytologist, although differentiating atypical transitional epithelial cells from dysplastic transitional epithelial cells is challenging when significant inflammation is present. In addition, cells may be in varying stages of deterioration which can exaggerate nuclear size and alter detail.

Next Steps

The presence of suspected neoplastic cells should be confirmed by a veterinary clinical pathologist/cytologist. Several stained and unstained smears of urine sediment, as well as fresh urine, should be submitted for evaluation. Air-dried, pre-made smears should be submitted as cells in fluid deteriorate quickly, which can hinder cytologic evaluation. A biopsy of the lesion for histologic examination may be needed to confirm a neoplastic process, distinguishing hyperplasia from malignancy (Figure 4.422).

If malignancy is confirmed, imaging (radiography, ultrasonography, computed tomography [CT], magnetic resonance imaging [MRI]) of the urinary system is recommended to locate the primary site. Surgery or appropriate chemotherapy or radiation therapy may be undertaken depending on the type and location of the neoplasm.

If malignancy is not confirmed, imaging (radiography, ultrasonography, CT, MR) of the urinary system is recommended to further characterize the lesion. An image-guided biopsy for histologic examination may be necessary to establish the nature of the lesion.

Figure 4.375 Urine from a dog. Aggregates of epithelial cells and RBCs (200×).

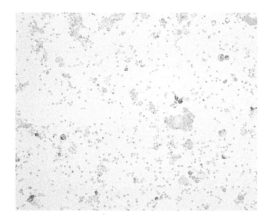

Figure 4.376 Hematuria and transitional cells (200×).

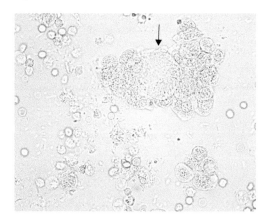

Figure 4.377 The cells, when examined with higher magnification, appear atypical; variation in cell size with a very large cell in the middle of the cell cluster (arrow). There are numerous WBCs and bacteria (500×).

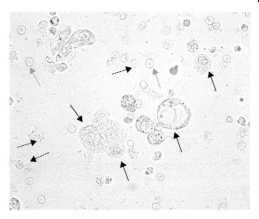

Figure 4.378 There is significant size variability among the transitional cells (arrows). WBCs (dashed arrows), RBCs (blue arrows), and bacteria in the background (500×).

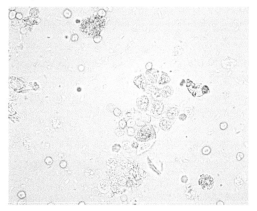

Figure 4.379 Neoplastic cells with prominent nucleus and size variability, RBCs, WBCs, and bacteria (500×).

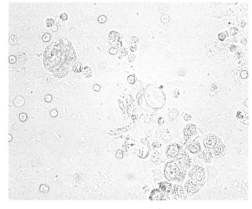

Figure 4.380 Large atypical cell with vacuole (center), large cell or tightly cohesive group of cells in upper left corner, and cells in the bottom right exhibiting variation in cell size. Some RBCs, WBCs, and bacteria in background (500×).

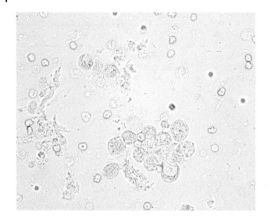

Figure 4.381 The cells are exhibiting variation in size. Some RBCs, WBCs, and bacteria in the background (500×).

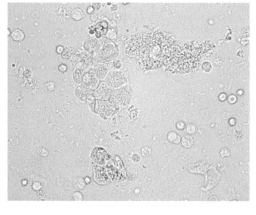

Figure 4.384 Transitional cells with prominent nuclear feature. Some RBCs, WBCs, and bacteria in the background; note the large aggregate of bacteria to the right of transitional cells (500×).

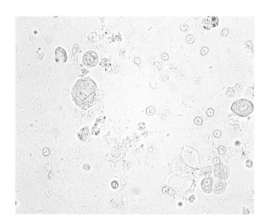

Figure 4.382 Large, atypical cell (upper left) and a group of transitional cells (lower right corner) with prominent nuclear features. RBCs, WBCs, and bacteria in the background (500×).

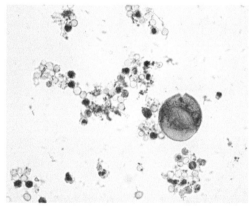

Figure 4.385 Urine from same dog as Figures 4.375–4.384. Large atypical cell with RBCs and WBCs in the background (supravital urine stain; 500×).

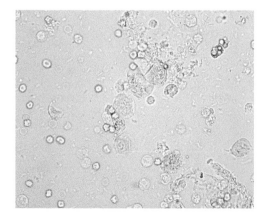

Figure 4.383 Transitional cells with prominent nuclear features and variation in cell size. Some RBCs, WBCs, and bacteria in the background (500×).

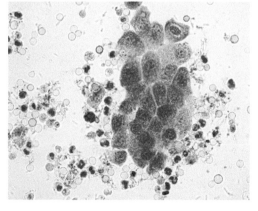

Figure 4.386 A sheet of transitional cells with variations in nuclear size (supravital urine stain; 500×)

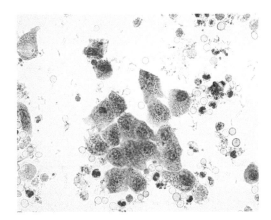

Figure 4.387 Group of transitional cells; cell in upper left corner has large vacuole that is displacing the nucleus (supravital urine stain; 500×).

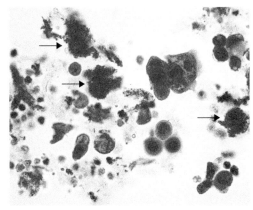

Figure 4.390 Individual transitional cells and a small group of transitional cells, and aggregates of bacteria (arrows) (supravital urine stain; 500×).

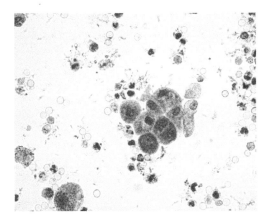

Figure 4.388 Transitional cells with variations in cell size, RBCs, WBCs, and bacteria (supravital urine stain; 500×).

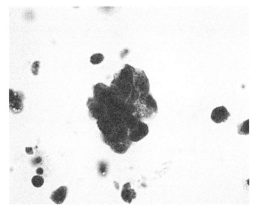

Figure 4.391 Cluster of transitional cells (supravital urine stain; 500×).

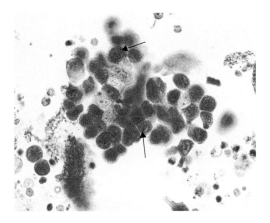

Figure 4.389 Group of transitional cells with variable cell size and variable nuclear size. The cells have prominent, often multiple nucleoli (arrows) (supravital urine stain; 500×).

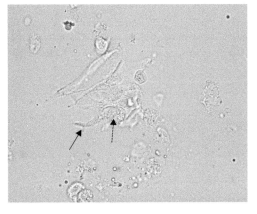

Figure 4.392 Urine from a cat with atypical epithelial cells. Some of the cells have tapering cytoplasm (arrow) and prominent internal features (dashed arrow) (500×).

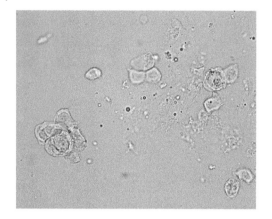

Figure 4.393 Cluster of atypical transitional cells with prominent internal features (500×).

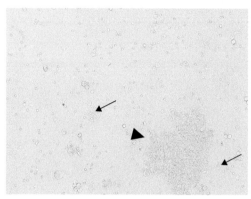

Figure 4.396 Disorganized group of epithelial cells (arrow head), variability in cell size, prominent nuclear features (arrows) (500×).

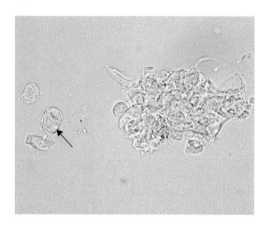

Figure 4.394 Disorganized cluster of epithelial cells; a cell with prominent vacuole (arrow) (500×).

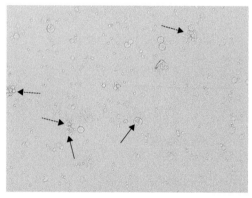

Figure 4.397 Transitional cells with prominent nuclear features (arrows) and disorganized groupings (dashed arrows) (500×).

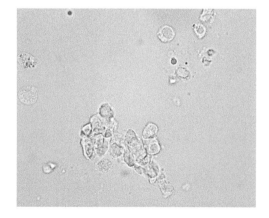

Figure 4.395 Group of epithelial cells with prominent internal features (500×).

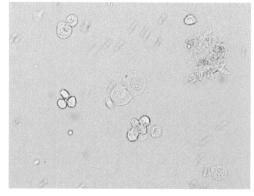

Figure 4.398 Transitional cells with prominent nuclear features (1000×).

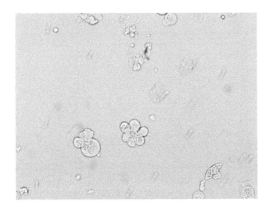

Figure 4.399 Transitional cells with prominent nuclear features and atypical arrangement (1000×).

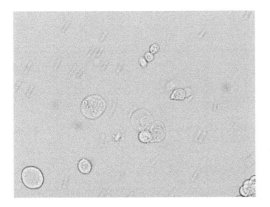

Figure 4.400 Transitional cells with prominent nuclear features (1000×).

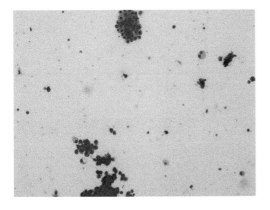

Figure 4.401 Urine from same cat as Figure 4.392–4.400. Moderately cellular preparation with clusters of transitional epithelial cells (Wright stain; 200×).

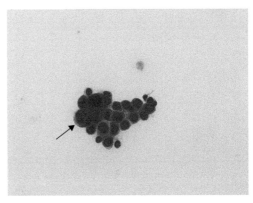

Figure 4.402 Cluster of epithelial cells with variable in nuclear size and high nuclear to cytoplasmic ratio. Variable nuclear size within one cell (arrow) (Wright stain; 500×).

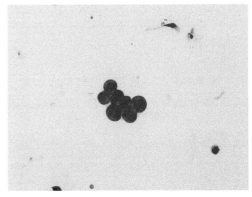

Figure 4.403 Group of epithelial cells (Wright stain; 500×).

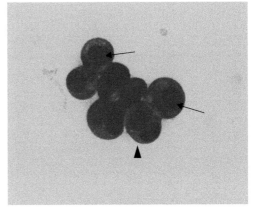

Figure 4.404 Group of epithelial cells with prominent nucleoli (arrows), binucleate cell (arrow head) (Wright stain; 1000×).

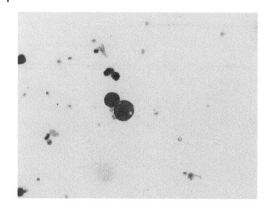

Figure 4.405 Neoplastic cells exhibiting variation in cell size and nuclear size, prominent nucleolus (Wright stain; 500×).

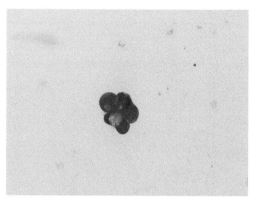

Figure 4.408 Tightly cohesive epithelial cells, one cell contains a vacuole that is displacing the nucleus (Wright stain; 500×).

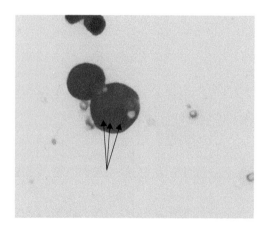

Figure 4.406 Neoplastic cells with coarse chromatin pattern, and three nucleoli (arrows) (Wright stain; 1000×).

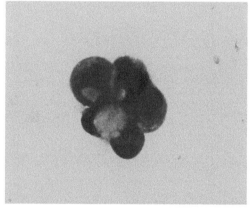

Figure 4.409 Tightly cohesive epithelial cells, one cell contains a vacuole that is displacing the nucleus (Wright stain; 1000×).

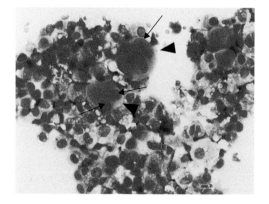

Figure 4.407 Neoplastic cells with variable nuclear sizes, multinucleated cells (arrow heads), prominent nucleoli (arrows) (Wright stain; 500×).

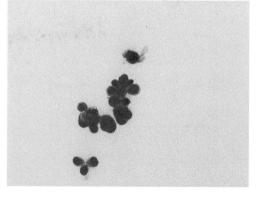

Figure 4.410 Neoplastic cells with a high nuclear to cytoplasmic ratio and coarse chromatin pattern (Wright stain; 500×).

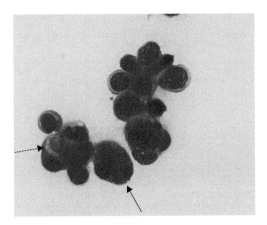

Figure 4.411 Neoplastic cells with a high nuclear to cytoplasmic ratio and coarse chromatin pattern. One cell contains a vacuole (dashed arrow); trinucleate cell (arrow) (Wright stain; 1000×).

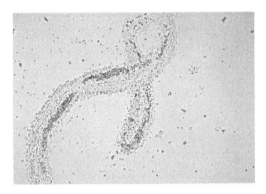

Figure 4.412 Urine from a dog with a mass-lesion in the trigone region of the urinary bladder. Large cast-like structure composed of transitional cells and RBCs (200×).

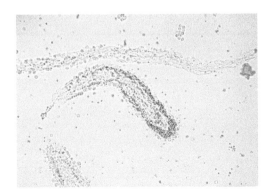

Figure 4.413 Large cast-like structures composed of transitional cells and RBCs (200×).

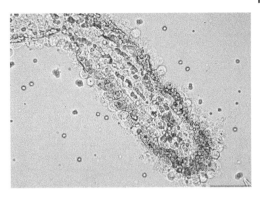

Figure 4.414 Large cast-like structure composed of transitional cells and RBCs (500×).

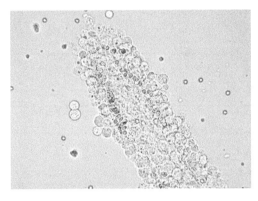

Figure 4.415 Large cast-like structures composed of transitional cells lining the outer perimeter and RBCs. The inner portion of this structure has a granular appearance with interspersed RBCs (500×).

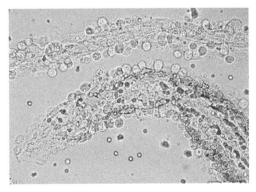

Figure 4.416 A large aggregate of transitional cells and RBCs (500×).

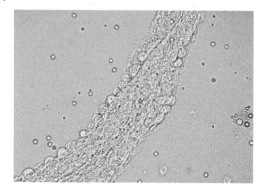

Figure 4.417 The inner area of this structure appears granular and individual cell detail is not clear. These cells may be deteriorating. Distinct cells are still visible lining the perimeter (500×).

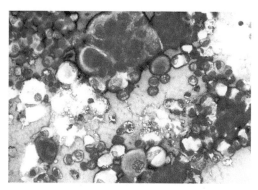

Figure 4.420 Clusters and individual cells exhibiting variation in nuclear size. A multinucleated cell is in the lower left corner (Wright stain; 500×).

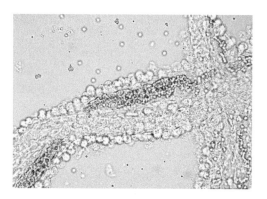

Figure 4.418 Intact cells are lining the perimeter, but the central area likely contains deteriorating cells. The RBCs may also be deteriorating in this section.

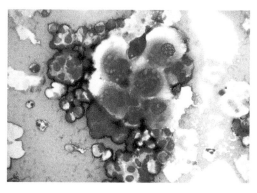

Figure 4.421 Clusters of cells exhibiting variation in nuclear size. A multinucleated cell is in the center group of large cells (Wright stain; 500×).

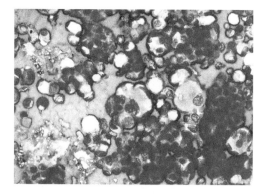

Figure 4.419 Urine from same dog as Figures 4.412–4.418. The sample is very cellular with many deteriorating epithelial cells, some in cohesive units, and RBCs in the background. (Wright stain; 500×).

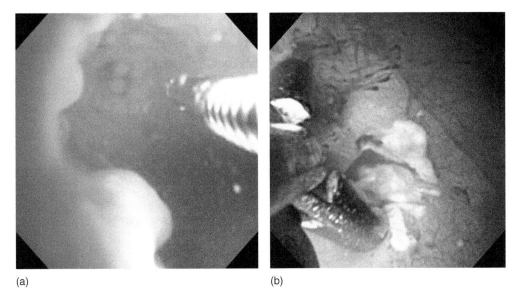

(a)   (b)

Figure 4.422 (a, b) The discovery of atypical cells on urinalysis may require biopsy and histopathology to determine if the cells are neoplastic and/or the type of neoplasia present. Endoscopic biopsies can sometimes be performed to confirm the presence of neoplasia.

Organisms

Organisms are occasionally found in urine sediment preparations. The discussion below covers most organisms that have been reported in urine preparations. Care must be taken not to misidentify artifacts as organisms. Some confusing artifacts are discussed in the "Miscellaneous Findings and Artifacts" section later in this chapter.

Bacteria

Distinctive Features
In unstained urine, bacterial rods are easier to differentiate from amorphous debris than are bacterial cocci (Figures 4.423–4.439). Occasionally bacteria in urine may appear filamentous or in chains that may branch. It is important to not confuse these with fungal hyphae. Fungal hyphae are usually larger in diameter. Bacteria amount is semi-quantitated typically using a 1+ (0–10 bacteria/hpf) to 5+ (>100 bacteria/hpf) scale.

Diagnostic Significance
Normally, urine in the bladder is sterile. Urine may become contaminated with bacteria as it passes from the bladder to the external environment. Bacterial contamination in voided or catheterized urine samples may not result in sufficient numbers of bacteria to be visualized microscopically in fresh urine samples. However, if the urine is allowed to sit at room temperature, bacterial numbers may increase sufficiently to be visualized microscopically. Urine that cannot be processed quickly should be refrigerated in a sealed container. Adding formalin decreases the potential for bacterial replication in stored urine. The urine sample may also be placed in a commercial preservative tube for anticipated culture and sensitivity (see Box 1.1).

The presence of high numbers of bacteria in fresh urine collected by catheterization or cystocentesis is suggestive of a urinary tract infection. There is typically a corresponding increase in WBCs (pyuria) present in the urine sediment along with the bacteria. High numbers of bacteria without pyuria suggest bacterial contamination, bacterial overgrowth due to time delay in evaluating the urine sample, or lysed WBCs. However, on occasion bacterial infections may occur with few WBC being present, especially in animals that are diabetic or immunosuppressed. Animals may have concurrent urinary tract or medical conditions which predispose them to infection, such as neoplasia, urolithiasis, structural or conformational defects, prolonged exposure to glucocorticoids (endogenous or exogenous), renal disease, or diabetes mellitus. Bacteria and WBCs may be shed intermittently in bacterial pyelonephritis.

Next Steps

Examiner error is a primary reason bacteria may be noted on examination of urine sediment but not confirmed by bacterial culture, especially when the urine sediment is unstained. If bacteria are seen in unstained urine sediment, confirm the presence of bacteria by evaluating an air-dried smear of urine sediment stained with a Romanowski-type rapid stain such as Diff-Quik. If bacteria are seen in stained urine sediment, the examiner may wish to rule out stain contamination by examining a cover-slipped slide containing a drop of stain without sediment. Urine culture should be performed periodically on patients with conditions predisposing to urinary tract infection such as hyperadrenocorticism, renal disease, and diabetes mellitus, even when bacteria and/or inflammatory cells are not observed on examination of urine sediment.

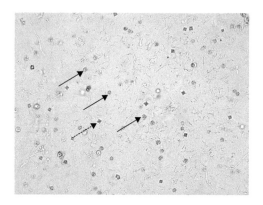

Figure 4.423 An abundant amount of bacterial rods with WBCs (arrows) and calcium oxalate dihydrate crystals (dashed arrow).

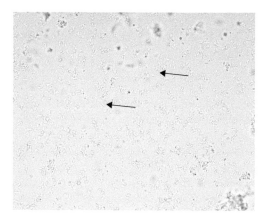

Figure 4.425 An abundant amount of bacteria and RBCs (arrows) (500×).

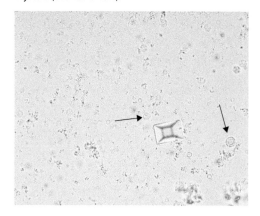

Figure 4.424 Urine from a cat. An abundant amount of bacterial cocci, WBCs (arrows), and a struvite crystal (500×).

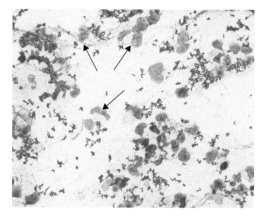

Figure 4.426 Urine from a cat. Degenerate cells and chromatin (arrows) and a large number of bacterial cocci (Wright stain; 500×).

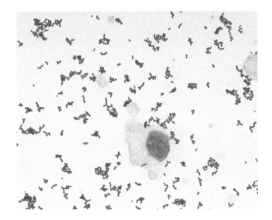

Figure 4.427 Bacterial cocci and a deteriorating cell (Wright stain; 1000×).

Figure 4.430 Moderately cellular urine sediment from a dog (100×).

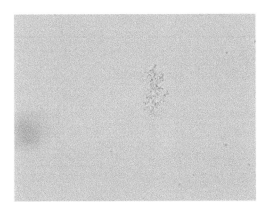

Figure 4.428 Urine from a dog. An aggregate of bacteria.

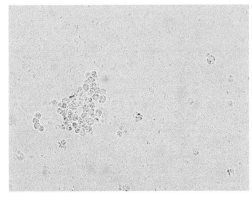

Figure 4.431 At higher magnification these cells can be identified as an aggregate of WBCs. An abundant amount of bacteria is present in the background (600×).

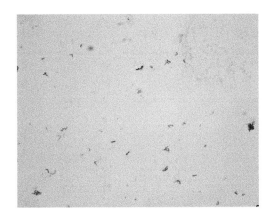

Figure 4.429 Bacterial rods (Wright stain; 1000×).

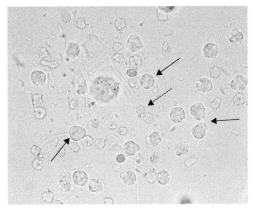

Figure 4.432 Moderate numbers of WBCs (arrows), RBCs (dashed arrow), and bacterial rods (600×).

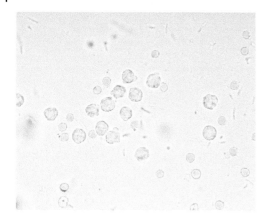

Figure 4.433 Moderate numbers of WBCs, RBCs, and bacterial rods (600×).

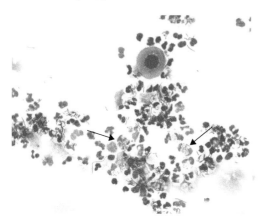

Figure 4.434 Degenerate neutrophils, some containing intracellular bacteria (arrows), a single transitional cell, and an abundant amount of background bacteria (Wright stain; 500×).

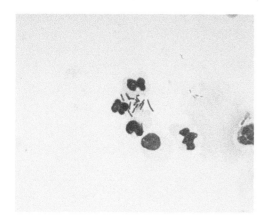

Figure 4.435 Degenerate neutrophils and bacterial rods (Wright stain; 500×).

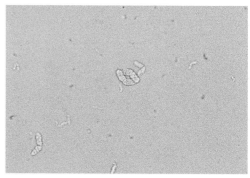

Figure 4.436 Urine from a dog. Unusual structures later identified as aggregates of bacteria (400×).

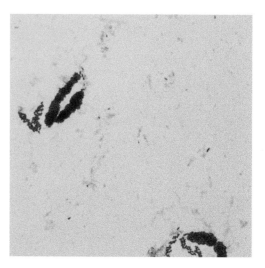

Figure 4.437 Aggregates of bacteria (Wright stain; 500×).

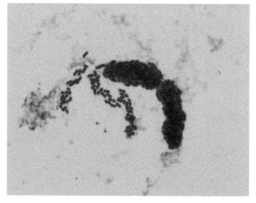

Figure 4.438 Aggregates of bacteria (Wright stain; 1000×).

Figure 4.439 Chains of bacterial cocci and calcium oxalate dihydrate crystals (500×).

Fungal Hyphae

Distinctive Features
Fungal hyphae may be septate (divisions between segments) or nonseptate (without segment division) and may, or may not, have terminal structures (Figures 4.440–4.448). Care should be taken to distinguish fungal hyphae from filamentous bacteria or chains of bacterial rods that can be branching. Bacteria are usually smaller in diameter.

Diagnostic Significance
Fungal hyphae and spores found in urinary sediment are often contaminants from the animal's hair, urine collection container, local environment, contaminated urine sediment stains, or skin of the person collecting the sample. Fungal infections of the urinary tract are uncommon, however *Candida* spp. is the most frequently reported. Most animals with *Candida* infection have predisposing concurrent urinary tract or medical conditions, such as prolonged antimicrobial use, prolonged exposure to glucocorticoids (endogenous or exogenous), renal disease, or diabetes mellitus.

Next Steps
Repeat the urinalysis with a fresh urine sample and confirm the presence of fungal organisms by evaluating an air-dried smear of urine sediment stained with a Romanowski-type rapid stain such as Diff-Quik. Submit an appropriately obtained urine sample for fungal culture. Fungal serology or antigen testing should be considered, if appropriate for the organism suspected. Review the patient's history and physical exam findings in addition to evaluating a CBC, biochemistry profile, and urine chemistry data to characterize any predisposing factors.

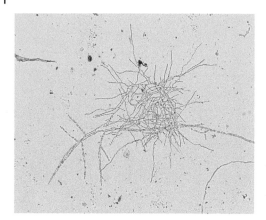

Figure 4.440 Contaminant branching fungal hyphae and a fungal spore (lower center). No inflammatory cells are evident (100×).

Figure 4.441 Contaminant branching fungal hyphae. No inflammatory cells are evident (100×).

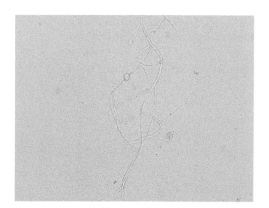

Figure 4.442 Contaminant branching fungal hyphae (200×).

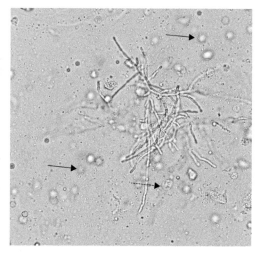

Figure 4.443 Urine from a dog with systemic aspergillosis. Branching fungal hyphae, RBCs (arrows), and WBCs (dashed arrow); the cells are in a different plane of focus (200×).

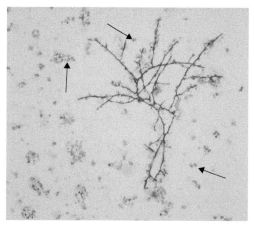

Figure 4.444 Urine from same dog as Figure 4.443. Branching fungal hyphae, scattered degenerate neutrophils (arrow), and RBCs (Wright stain; 500×).

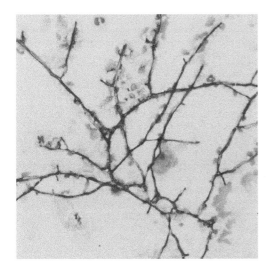

Figure 4.445 Urine from same dog as Figure 4.443. Branching fungal hyphae, scattered degenerate neutrophils, and RBCs (Wright stain; 1000×).

Figure 4.447 Contaminant fungal element; no inflammatory cells are evident (image from IDEXX SediVue Dx™ Urine Sediment Analyzer).

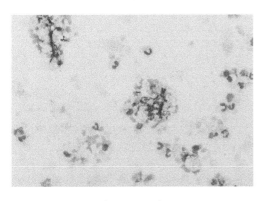

Figure 4.446 Urine from same dog as Figure 4.443. Branching fungal hyphae surrounded by degenerate neutrophils (Wright stain; 500×).

Figure 4.448 Contaminant fungal element; no inflammatory cells are evident (image from IDEXX SediVue Dx™ Urine Sediment Analyzer").

Yeast

Distinctive Features

Yeast organisms are small, round to ovoid, may be budding, and are refractive (Figures 4.449–4.453). Yeast must be distinguished from RBCs and fat droplets. Fat droplets may be of varying size and may stick together and resemble budding yeasts. Yeast are more variable in size and more refractive than RBCs. Fat droplets, like air bubbles, will float up under the coverslip and be in a different plane of focus if the sample is given several minutes to settle.

Diagnostic Significance

Yeast organisms are generally considered artifacts that occur in aged urine. Rarely, a pathogenic systemic mycotic organism such as *Blastomyces*, *Cryptococcus*, or *Candida* spp. colonizes the urinary or genital tract and may be found in urine. These pathogenic organisms are often accompanied by WBCs.

Next Steps

Same as for fungal hyphae.

Figure 4.449 Urine from a cat with moderate numbers of yeast (200×).

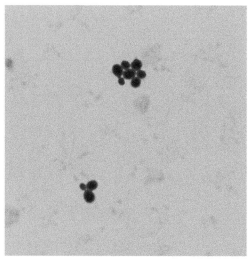

Figure 4.452 Urine from a dog with *Candida* sp. pyelonephritis (Wright stain; 1000×).

Figure 4.450 Budding yeast (200×).

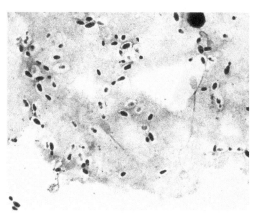

Figure 4.453 Urine from a dog. Budding yeast, sperm (urine stain; 1000×).

Figure 4.451 Varying sizes of budding yeast (*Cryptococcus* sp.) (400×).

Dioctophyma renale Ova

Distinctive Features

Dioctophyma renale eggs are oval and have thick, pitted shells except at their poles (Figures 4.454–4.458). Hematuria and/or pyuria may also be observed in the urine sediment of infected dogs.

Diagnostic Significance

Rarely, dogs may become parasitized with *Dioctophyma renale* through consumption of infected fish or frogs. After ingestion, *Dioctophyma* larvae penetrate the duodenum and migrate through the peritoneum to the kidney where they mature. The predilection for the right kidney is presumed to be due to the proximity of the right kidney to the duodenum; however the nematode can encyst anywhere in the abdominal cavity. Detection of *Dioctophyma renale* eggs in the urine indicates that a gravid female is present in the urinary excretory tract of the animal.

Next Steps

Imaging studies (radiography, ultrasonography, MRI) are useful in determining parasite location. Nephrectomy is often recommended if one kidney is involved.

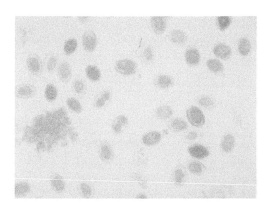

Figure 4.454 *Dioctophyma renale* ova (100×).

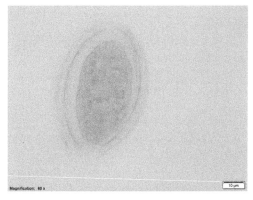

Figure 4.456 *Dioctophyma renale* ova (600×).

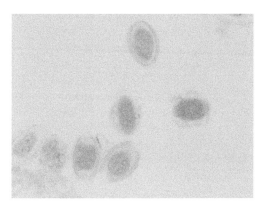

Figure 4.455 *Dioctophyma renale* ova (200×).

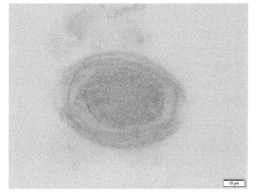

Figure 4.457 *Dioctophyma renale* ova have pitted shells except at their poles (600×).

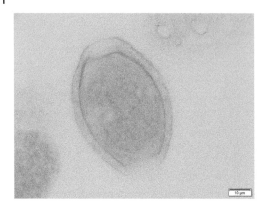

Figure 4.458 *Dioctophyma renale* ova (600×).

Capillaria plica (now Pearsonema plica) and Capillaria felis cati Ova

Distinctive Features
Capillaria (Pearsonema) plica and *Capillaria felis cati* eggs are colorless and oval with a slightly pitted surface and bipolar plugs (Figures 4.459–4.466). They must be distinguished from *Trichuris vulpis* eggs, which may be found in voided urine samples due to fecal contamination. Hematuria, pyuria, and increased numbers of transitional cells may be observed in the urine sediment of *Capillaria*-infected dogs or cats. Although most cats and dogs are asymptomatic, some may experience pollakiuria, urinary incontinence, and inappropriate urination. Affected cats could experience abdominal pain, fever, distended painful urinary bladder, and urinary blockage.

Adult *Capillaria* may be found in urine sediment. They are small threadlike, yellowish parasites 13–60 mm long.

Diagnostic Significance
Finding *Capillaria* eggs or adults indicates infection. *C. (P.) plica* is usually found in the urinary bladder and, less commonly, in the renal pelves and ureters of dogs, and *C. felis cati* is the parasite usually found in the urinary bladder of the cat. These two species are similar in most respects and are transmitted to their respective hosts by ingestion of earthworms that contain the first-stage larvae. The larvae migrate from the intestine to the urinary bladder where they are embedded in the urinary bladder epithelium.

Next Steps
Evaluate the infected animal's condition in accordance with the patient's clinical signs and treat appropriately. The majority of infected cats and dogs are asymptomatic, and *Capillaria* eggs are discovered in urine sediment incidentally. Preventing cats and dogs from ingesting earthworms may not only prevent initial *Capillaria* infection but also play a primary role in the elimination of *Capillaria* from infected animals, since evidence exists that capillariasis may be a self-limiting disease when re-infection does not occur (Waddell, 1968). Reported treatments include levamisole, fenbendazole, albendazole, and ivermectin.

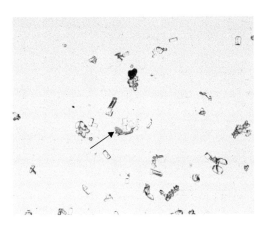

Figure 4.459 Urine from a cat. A single *Pearsonema plica* ova (arrow) amongst struvite crystals (100×).

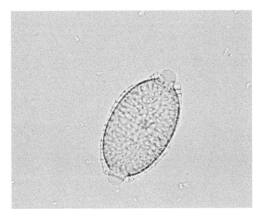

Figure 4.462 *Pearsonema plica* ova are oval with pitted surface and bipolar plugs (1000×).

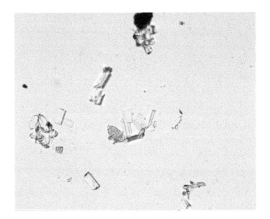

Figure 4.460 *Pearsonema plica* ova (200×).

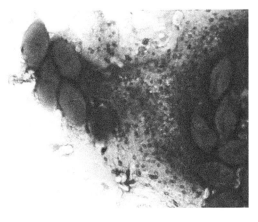

Figure 4.463 *Pearsonema plica* ova (Wright stain; 500×).

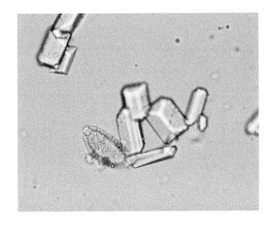

Figure 4.461 *Pearsonema plica* ova (500×).

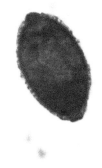

Figure 4.464 *Pearsonema plica* ova (Wright stain; 1000×).

Figure 4.465 Urine from a dog. *Pearsonema plica* ova (400×).

Figure 4.466 *Pearsonema plica* ova (400×).

Microfilaria

Distinctive Features
Dirofilaria immitis microfilariae are occasionally found in urine sediment (Figures 4.467–4.470). Their presence in urine is presumably due to hemorrhage into the excretory pathway of the urinary system. They are 307–322 μm long and 6–7 μm wide. *D. immitis* microfilariae have a straight posterior end and tapering anterior end.

Diagnostic Significance
Indicates heartworm infection.

Next Steps
If desired, *Dirofilaria immitis* antigen testing may be performed to confirm the diagnosis. Additional evaluation of the infected animal's condition should be performed, including a CBC, biochemistry profile, and thoracic radiography, followed by appropriate treatment.

Figure 4.467 Urine from a dog. Hematuria with a single microfilaria (100×).

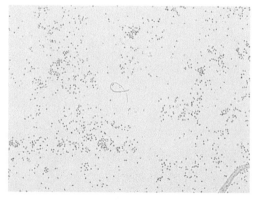

Figure 4.468 Hematuria with a single microfilaria (100×).

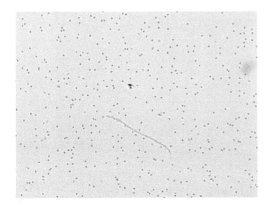

Figure 4.469 Hematuria with a single microfilaria (200×).

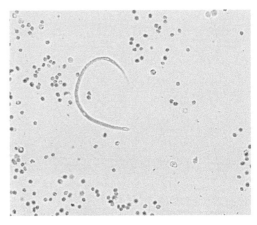

Figure 4.470 Hematuria with a single microfilaria (400×).

Miscellaneous Findings and Artifacts

Pollen

Distinctive Features
Pollen grains are generally round to oval in form, may have a yellow to brown tint, and can sometimes have a small stem that aids in their identification (Figures 4.471–4.474).

Diagnostic Significance
Free-catch urine samples may contain pollen grains which may be misidentified as parasite eggs or bizarre crystals. Familiarity with the features of parasites and crystals that may appear in the urine, and limiting contamination of urine samples will decrease the likelihood of confusing pollen grains with other structures.

Next Steps
If concern remains that the observed structure is something other than a pollen grain or other harmless contaminant, the examiner should consider consulting a veterinary clinical pathologist and submitting an air-dried smear of urine sediment containing the structure(s), if possible, for further evaluation.

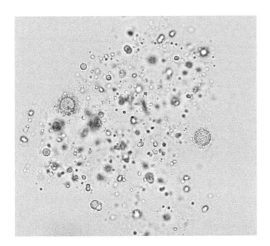

Figure 4.471 Urine from a dog. Two pollen structures; these can be misidentified as parasite ova (200×).

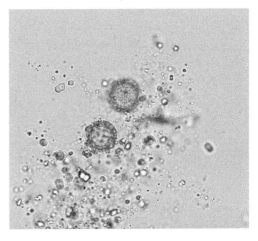

Figure 4.472 Pollen: thick-walled and pitted surface (400×).

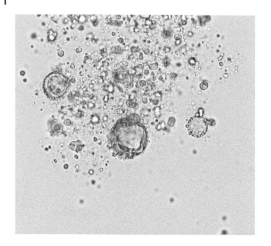

Figure 4.473 Pollen (400×).

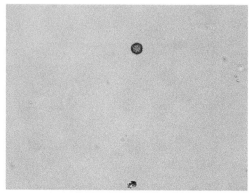

Figure 4.474 Pollen (image from IDEXX SediVue Dx™ Urine Sediment Analyzer).

Fungal Spores

Distinctive Features
Fungal spores are generally round, oval, or oblong in form, may have a yellow to brown tint, and can sometimes have internal septae (Figures 4.475–4.483).

Diagnostic Significance
Free-catch urine samples may contain non-pathogenic fungal spores which may be misidentified as parasite eggs or bizarre crystals. Familiarity with the features of parasites and crystals that may appear in the urine, and limiting contamination of urine samples will decrease the likelihood of confusing fungal spores with other structures.

Next Steps
If concern remains that the observed structure is something other than a nonpathogenic fungal spore or other harmless contaminant, the examiner should consider consulting a veterinary clinical pathologist and submitting an air-dried smear of urine sediment containing the structure(s), if possible, for further evaluation.

Figure 4.475 Fungal spore (*Altenaria*) (100×).

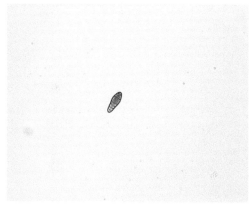

Figure 4.476 Fungal spore (200×).

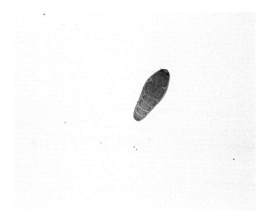

Figure 4.477 Fungal spore (500×).

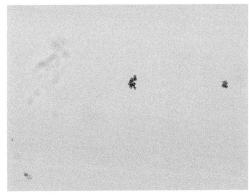

Figure 4.480 Urine from a dog. Fungal spores (100×).

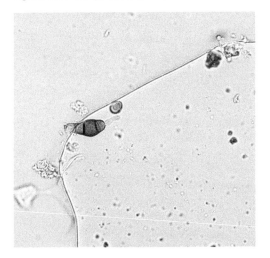

Figure 4.478 Fungal spore (400×).

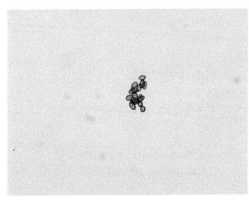

Figure 4.481 Fungal spores (200×).

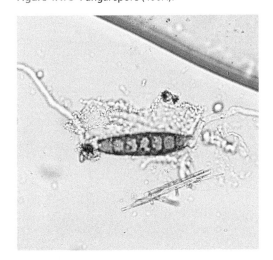

Figure 4.479 Fungal spore (600×).

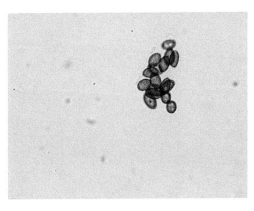

Figure 4.482 Fungal spores (600×).

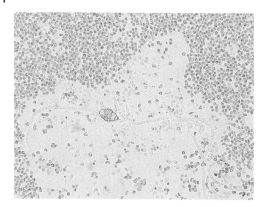

Figure 4.483 Germinating fungal spore, hematuria (400×).

Mucus

Distinctive Features
Mucus strands are long, thin structures with a low refractive index in unstained urine (Figures 4.484–4.486). In stained urine, mucus and mucus strands frequently stain very dark and may obstruct visualization of other urine sediment components. Therefore, urine sediment containing abundant mucus often must be evaluated unstained.

Diagnostic Significance
Strands of mucus can be misidentified as granular or hyaline casts, adult *Capillaria*, or microfilariae. When compared with casts, mucus strands tend to be more irregular in shape and often have tapered ends. Mucus strands occasionally occur in urine of dog and cats and usually are associated with inflammation of the urogenital tract.

Next Steps
Assess the patient's urine for other evidence of urinary tract inflammation to help confirm that the observed structures are likely composed of mucus and to evaluate the need for further diagnostic procedures.

Figure 4.484 Mucus (image from IDEXX SediVue Dx™ Urine Sediment Analyzer).

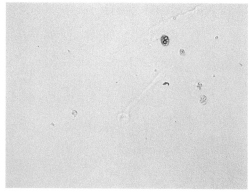

Figure 4.485 Mucus (image from IDEXX SediVue Dx™ Urine Sediment Analyzer).

Figure 4.486 Mucus (image from IDEXX SediVue Dx™ Urine Sediment Analyzer).

Lipid Droplets

Distinctive Features

Lipid droplets are variably sized, spherical structures with smooth outer contours. They have a different (higher) refractive index than urine causing them to refract light and "glisten" (Figures 4.487–4.491). Also, they are lighter than urine and therefore float and are in a different plane of focus than the remainder of the urine sediment. These features allow them to be differentiated from RBCs, parasite eggs, yeast, etc.

Diagnostic Significance

Urine sediment from cats or diabetic dogs often contains fat droplets. This is likely due to the lipid content of their renal tubular cells.

Next Steps

None required, generally an incidental finding.

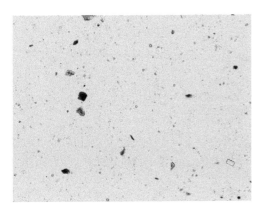

Figure 4.487 Lipid droplets are variably sized, round structures that are refractile (100×).

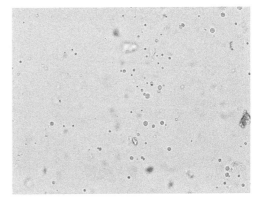

Figure 4.488 Lipid droplets (200×).

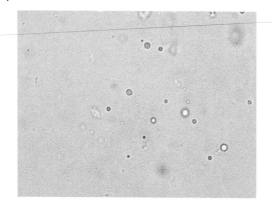

Figure 4.489 Lipid droplets (500×).

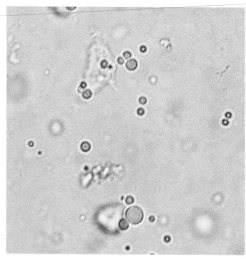

Figure 4.491 Lipid droplets (1000×).

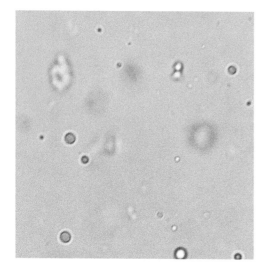

Figure 4.490 Lipid droplets (1000×).

Sperm

Distinctive Features

Spermatozoa have oval heads and long, thin tails (Figures 4.492–4.498).

Diagnostic Significance

Spermatozoa may be an incidental finding in urine from intact males, including urine collected by cystocentesis. Occasionally, sperm may be found in free-catch urine samples from females post breeding.

Next Steps

None required.

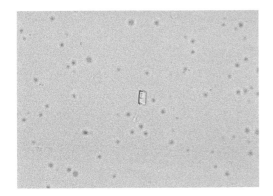

Figure 4.492 Sperm and struvite crystal (200×).

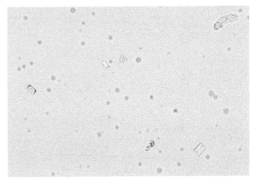

Figure 4.495 Sperm and struvite crystals (200×).

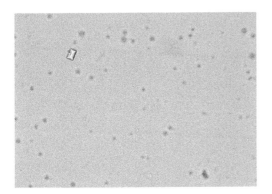

Figure 4.493 Sperm and struvite crystal (200×).

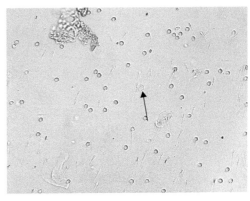

Figure 4.496 Numerous sperm, RBCS, and one WBC (arrow) (image from IDEXX SediVue Dx™ Urine Sediment Analyzer).

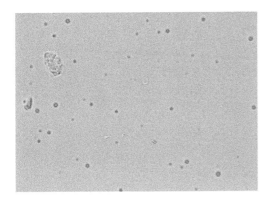

Figure 4.494 Sperm (200×).

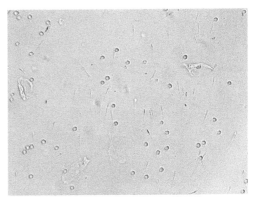

Figure 4.497 Numerous sperm, RBCs, and squamous epithelial cells (image from IDEXX SediVue Dx™ Urine Sediment Analyzer).

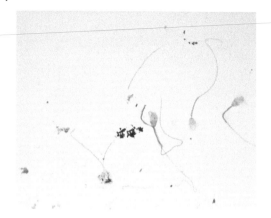

Figure 4.498 Sperm (Wright stain; 1000×).

Air Bubbles

Distinctive Features

Like fat droplets, air bubbles exist in a different plane of focus than the rest of the urine sediment if sufficient time is given before microscopic evaluation. Unlike fat, air bubbles appear flat, instead of spherical, and do not glisten (Figures 4.499–4.501).

Diagnostic Significance

Air bubbles occur when air is trapped between the coverslip and urine sediment as the coverslip is placed over the urine sediment.

Next Steps

None required.

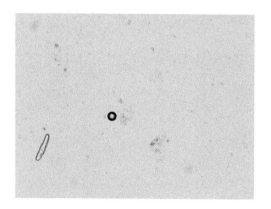

Figure 4.499 Air bubble (100×).

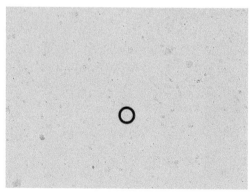

Figure 4.500 Air bubble (200×).

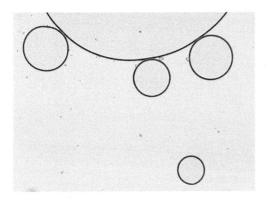

Figure 4.501 Air bubbles (100×).

Starch Granules (Glove Powder)

Distinctive Features
Starch granules or crystals are clear granules with a central fissure with borders which are commonly hexagonal in shape but which may take on a rounder appearance (Figures 4.502–4.505). Under polarized light these crystals will appear as "Maltese crosses".

Diagnostic Significance
Starch granules in urine sediment are considered an incidental finding, resulting from contamination of urine samples with examination glove powder used in urine collection (Figure 4.506).

Next Steps
None required.

Figure 4.502 Numerous starch granules (glove powder) (100×).

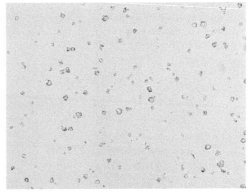

Figure 4.503 Glove powder (200×).

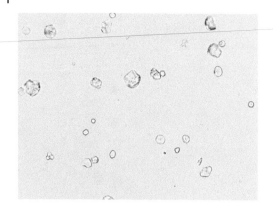

Figure 4.504 Glove powder (500×).

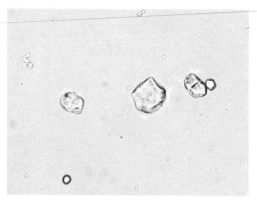

Figure 4.505 Glove powder (1000×).

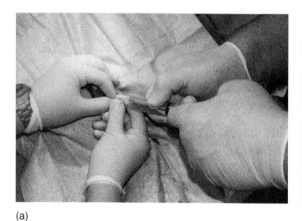

(a)

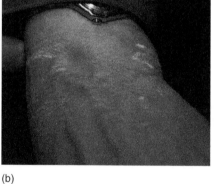

(b)

Figure 4.506 (a) Surgical and examination gloves are a potential source of contamination of urine samples with starch granules. (b) Glove powder can be seen on the wrist of this individual after wearing surgical gloves and could potentially contaminate a urine sample with starch granules.

Fiber

Distinctive Features

Fibers are typically linear structures that can have variable margins (Figures 4.507–4.509).

Diagnostic Significance

Fibers in urine sediment are considered an incidental finding, resulting from contamination of the urine sample.

Next Steps

None required.

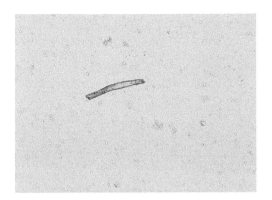

Figure 4.507 Fiber (200×).

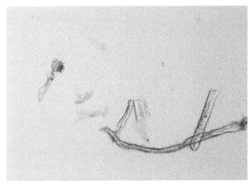

Figure 4.509 Fiber and debris (200×).

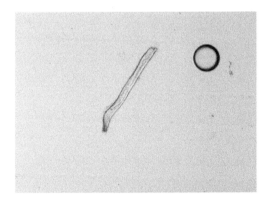

Figure 4.508 Fiber and air bubble (200×).

References

Adams LG and Syme HM. (2010) Canine ureteral and lower urinary tract diseases. In: *Textbook of Veterinary Internal Medicine* 7th edn, Ettinger SJ and Feldman EC eds. St. Louis, MO: Saunders, pp. 2086–2115.

Bartges JW. (2005) Discolored urine. In: *Textbook of Veterinary Internal Medicine* 6th edn, Ettinger SJ and Feldman EC eds. St. Louis, MO: Elsevier, pp. 112–114.

Bowles M. (2008) The diagnostic approach to hematuria. *Veterinary Medicine* 103(7): 374–391.

Bowles MH and Lorenz MD (2009) *Small Animal Medical Diagnosis* 3rd edn. Ames, IO: Wiley-Blackwell, pp. 258–273.

Davies C and Shell L. (2002) *Common Small Animal Diagnoses: An Alogrithmic Approach.* Philadelphia, PA: Saunders, p. 201.

Feldman EC and Nelson RW. (2004) Canine diabetes mellitus. In: *Canine and Feline Endocrinology and Reproduction.* St. Louis, MO: Elsevier, p. 491.

Fry MM. (2011) Urinalysis. In: *Nephrology and Urology of Small Animals*, Bartges J and Polzin DJ eds. Ames, IO: Wiley-Blackwell, pp. 46–57.

George JW. (2001) The usefulness and limitations of hand-held refractometers in veterinary laboratory medicine: an historical and technical review. *Veterinary Clinical Pathology* 30(4): 201–210.

Hoenig M, Dorfman M, and Koenig A. (2008) Use of a hand-held meter for the measurement of blood beta-hydroxybutyrate in dogs and cats. *Journal of Veterinary Emergency and Critical Care* 18: 86–87.

Johnson KY, Lulich JP, and Osborne CA. (2007) Evaluation of the reproducibility and accuracy of pH-determining devices used to measure urine pH in dogs. *Journal of the American Veterinary Medical Association* 230(3): 364–369.

Laffel L. (1999) A review of physiology, pathophysiology and application of monitoring to diabetes. *Diabetes/ Metabolism Research and Reviews* 15: 412–426.

Lees GE, Jensen WA, Sipson DF, et al. (2002) Persistent albuminuria precedes onset of overt proteinuria in male dogs with with X-linked hereditary nephropathy. *Journal of Veterinary Internal Medicine* 16: 353.

Lulich JP and Osborne CA. (1999) Bacterial urinary tract infections. In: *Textbook of Veterinary Internal Medicine* 4th edn, Ettinger SJ and Feldman EC eds. Philadelphia, PA: WB Saunders, pp. 1775–1788.

Mahmud N, Stinson J, O'Connell MA, et al. (1994) Microalbuminuria in inflammatory bowel disease. *Gut* 35: 1599–1604.

Nelson RW and Couto CG. (2003) Lymphadenopathy and splenomegaly. In: *Small Animal Internal Medicine* 3rd edn. St. Louis, MO: Mosby, pp. 1200–1209.

Osborne CA, Bartger JW, Lulich JP. (2004) Feline xanthine urolithiasis: a newly recognized cause of urinary tract disease. *Urological Research* 32(2): 171 (abstract).

Atlas of Canine and Feline Urinalysis, First Edition. Theresa E. Rizzi, Amy Valenciano, Mary Bowles, Rick Cowell, Ronald Tyler, and Dennis B. DeNicola.
© 2017 John Wiley & Sons, Inc. Published 2017 by John Wiley & Sons, Inc.

Osborne CA, Stevens JB. (1999) Biochemical analysis of urine: Indications, methods, interpretation. In: *Urinalysis: A Clinical Guide to Compassionate Patient Care.* Robinson, PA: Veterinary Learning Systems, p. 100.

Pedersen LM and Milman N. (1998) Microalbuminuria in patients with lung cancer. *European Journal of Cancer* 34: 76–80.

Pressler BM, Vaden SL, and Jensen W. (2001) Prevalence of microalbuminuria in dogs evaluated at a referral veterinary hospital. *Journal of Veterinary Internal Medicine* 15: 300.

Stojanovic V and Ihle S. (2011) Role of beta-hydroxybutyric acid in diabetic ketoacidosis: a review. *Canadian Veterinary Journal* 52(4): 426–430.

Tommaso M, Aste G, Rocconi F, et al. (2009) Evaluation of a portable meter to measure ketonemia and comparison with ketonuria for the diagnosis of canine diabetic ketoacidosis. *Journal of Veterinary Internal Medicine* 23: 466–471.

Vaden SL, Jensen W, Longhofer S, et al. (2001) Longitudinal study of microalbuminuria in soft-coated wheaten terriers. *Journal of Veterinary Internal Medicine* 2001; 15: 300 (abstract).

Waddell AH. (1968) Further observations on *Capillaria feliscati* in the cat. *Australian Veterianry Journal* 44: 33–34.

Welles E, Whatley E, Hall A, et al. (2006) Comparison of Multistix PRO dipsticks with other biochemical assays for determining urine protein (UP), urine creatinine (UC), and UP:UC ratio in dogs and cats. *Veterinary Clinical Pathology* 35: 31–36.

Whittemore JC, Gill VL, Jensen WA, et al. (2006) Evaluation of the association between microalbuminuria and the urine albumin-creatinine ratio and systemic disease in dogs. *Journal of the American Veterinary Medical Association* 229: 958–963.

Whittemore JC, Miyoshi Z, Jensen WA, et al. (2007) Association of microalbuminuria and the urine albumin-to-creatinine ratio with systemic disease in cats. *Journal of the American Veterinary Medical Association* 230: 1165–1169.

Zeugswetter F and Pagitz M. (2009) Ketone measurements using dipstick methodology in cats with diabetes mellitus. *Journal of Small Animal Practice* 50: 4–8.

Index

Note: Page numbers followed by t, f, and b indicate tables, figures, and boxes, respectively.

a

Acetest™   62
air bubbles   176, 176f–177f, 179f
albumin   54–56, 55t
algorithm, for red or brown urine   49
amyloidosis   57t
artifacts, in urine samples   169

b

bacteria, in urine   157–158, 158f–161f
BD Vacutainer®   4b, 5f
Bence-Jones protein   54, 55t, 56, 60
bilirubin   64–65, 64t–65t
blood   63–65, *see* hematuria

c

Capillaria plica, see Pearsonema plica
casts   67–68
   cellular   71–72, 73f
   fatty   79, 79f–81f
   fine granular   77f
   granular   73–74, 74f–77f
   hemoglobin   81, 81f–82f
   hyaline   68, 69–71f
   leukocyte   71–72
   lipid, *see* fatty
   mixed   82, 82f–84f
   pseudo   85, 85f
   red blood cell   71–72, 73f

waxy   78, 78f–79f
white blood cell, *see* leukocyte
catheterization, transurethral   15–18
   blind, female   33b, 36f–37f
   digital, female   17–18, 31b, 32f
   equipment, (canine)   27f, (feline)   30f, 37f
   visualization, female   17, 23b, (canine)   23b–24b, 28f–29f, (feline)   24b–25b, 30f
   visualization, male   18b–19b, 21f–22f
catheters, urinary   15–17, 16f
   determining length   20f, 26f
chemistry, urine   53. *See also* individual tests
clarity, urine physical characteristics   43
concentrating ability   50
   interference   50, 50t
crystals, urine   84
   ammonium urate (biurate)   104, 104f–109f
   amorphous   117–118, 118f–119f
   ampicillin   131
   bilirubin   120, 121f–126f
   calcium oxalate dihydrate   93, 93f–96f

calcium oxalate monohydrate   96, 97f–101f
   calcium phosphate   102, 102f–103f
   cholesterol   128, 129f
   cystine   111, 112f–117f
   leucine   120
   melamine, melamine cyanurate   127, 127f–128f
   radiopaque contrast   128
   struvite   86, 86f–90f
      dissolving   89f–92f
   sulfonamide (sulfa)   130, 130f–131f
   triple phosphate, *see* struvite
   tyrosine   120
   urate, *see* ammonium urate
   uric acid   109, 109f–111f
   xanthine   117
culture, urine   44–46, 156
culture preservative tube   4b, 5f
cystocentesis   37–38, 39b
   bladder palpation   42f, 44f
   equipment   37, 38f
   ultrasound guided   40b, 42f–44f

d

Dioctophyma renale ova   165, 165f–166f
dipstick colorimetric test (DSCT)   53, 54f

Atlas of Canine and Feline Urinalysis, First Edition. Theresa E. Rizzi, Amy Valenciano, Mary Bowles, Rick Cowell, Ronald Tyler, and Dennis B. DeNicola.
© 2017 John Wiley & Sons, Inc. Published 2017 by John Wiley & Sons, Inc.

e

EDTA tube   4t, 5f
epithelial cells, *see* individual
     type
erythrocytes, in urine, *see*
     hematuria

f

false negative, protein   56t
false positive, protein   56t
fiber, in urine   178, 179f
free catch urine collection   3,
     4b, 9b, 13b, 14f
   equipment   4f–5f, 7f, 9f,
     15f
fungal hyphae, in urine   161,
     162f–163f
fungal spores, in urine   170,
     170f–172f

g

glomerular, causes of
     proteinuria   55t
glomerular filtration rate
     (GFR)   56
glomerulonephritis   57t
glove powder   177, 177f–178f
glucose   60–61

h

hematuria   47, 49t, 63, 64t,
     143, 145–146,
     146f–148f
hemoglobin, urine chemistry
     55, 49f, 55t, 63–64, 64t,
     65
Heska's ERDScreen™ Urine
     Test   57
hyposthenuria   50

i

isosthenuria   50

k

ketones   61–62
ketonometer   62, 62f

l

leukocytes (WBCs), in urine
     141, 141f–143f

degenerate neutrophils
     144f–145f
lipid droplets   173, 173f–174f

m

microalbuminuria (MA)
     test   57–60
microfilaria, in urine   168,
     168f–170f
mucus   172, 172f–173f
myoglobin, urine chemistry
     54, 49f, 55t, 63
   myoglobinuria   63, 64t

n

neoplasia   148, 149f–156f
   endoscopic biopsy   157f
nonabsorbent beads   15f

o

odor, urine   48
osmolality, urine   49
output, urine   50

p

Pearsonema plica ova   166,
     167f–168f
pH, urine
   changes in   54
   measurement   53–54
   range   54
pollen   169, 169f–170f
polydypsia   50t
polyuria   50t
post-void urine collection
     4–5, 13b, 14f–15f
protein, in urine   54–60,
     55t–57t, 59t
   and pH   54
   and specific gravity   55

q

quantitative measure, urine
     protein   56

r

red blood cells, in urine, *see*
     hematuria
refractometer   50–51, 49f
renal tubular cells   140
   in casts   71

s

sediment, urine   67
specific gravity, urine   49–51
sperm   174, 175f–176f
squamous cells, in urine   136,
     137f–139f
   bilirubin stained   140f
starch granules   177, *see*
     glove powder
sulfosalicylic acid (SSA)
     turbidity test   55
supravital stains   67

t

Tamm–Horsfall mucoprotein
     68, 71, 78
transitional cells   131–132,
     132f–135f
   deteriorating   135f–136f
   neoplastic   148, 149f–156f
transurethral catheterization
     15–17
   blind, female   33b, 36f–37f
   digital, female   17–18, 31b,
     32f
     equipment, (canine)   27f,
     (feline)   30f, 37f
   visualization, female   17,
     23b,
     (canine)   23b–24b,
     28f–29f,
     (feline)   24b–25b, 30f
   visualization, male   18b,
     21f–22f
turbidity, urine physical
     characteristics   43

u

urine
   changes with delay   44,
     45b
   chemistry   53
   clarity   48, 49f
   collection   3
     amount   4b, 4f
     general principles   4b
     manual expression   9b,
     11f–12f
     normal void   6b, 7f–8f,
     9b

color   47–48, 48f–49f
containers   4b, 5f, 7f–8f
    homemade devices   7f
mid-stream collection   3
normal output   47
sediment preparation
    67

urine protein/creatinine ratio
    55, 58
    interpretation   57t–58t,
        59t

v
volume, for examination   67

w
white blood cells (WBCs), *see*
    leukocytes
Wright stain   67

y
yeast   163, 164f